Caregiving *in*
The Comfort of Home®

4TH EDITION

A Complete Guide for Caregivers

Caregiving in The Comfort of Home® caregiver book series is written for family and paraprofessional home caregivers who face the resposibilities of caring for aging friends, family, or clients. The disease-specific editions, often in collaboration with organizations supporting those conditions, address caregivers assisting people with those diseases.

Other Caregiver Resources from CareTrust Publications:

La comodidad del hogar® *(Spanish Edition)*
The Comfort of Home® *Multiple Sclerosis Edition*
The Comfort of Home ® *for Parkinson Disease*
The Comfort of Home ® *for Stroke*
The Comfort of Home ® *for Alzheimer's Disease*
The Comfort of Home® *for Chronic Lung Disease*
The Comfort of Home® *for Chronic Liver Disease*
The Comfort of Home® *for Chronic Heart Failure*
The Comfort of Home ® *Caregiving Journal*
The Comfort of Home ® *Caregivers—Let's Take Care of You!* Meditation CD

Newsletters:

The Comfort of Home® *Caregiver Assistance News*
The Comfort of Home® *Grand-Parenting News*
The Comfort of Home® *Caregivers—Let's Take Care of You!*

Visit *www.comfortofhome.com* for forthcoming editions and other caregiver resources.

Caregiving in
The Comfort of Home®

4TH EDITION

A Complete Guide for Caregivers

Maria M. Meyer

and

Paula Derr, RN, BSN, CEN, CCRN

CareTrust Publications LLC
"Caring for you... caring for others."
Portland, Oregon

Caregiving in The Comfort of Home®: A Complete Guide for Caregivers

This book is updated from the previously published edition as *The Comfort of Home®: A Complete Guide for Caregivers* Third Edition.

Published by: CareTrust Publications LLC
P.O. Box 10283
Portland, Oregon 97296-0283
(800) 565-1533
Fax (415) 673-2205

Publisher's Cataloging-in-Publication
(Provided by Quality Books, Inc.)

Meyer, Maria M., 1948-
 [Comfort of home]
 Caregiving in the comfort of home: a complete guide
for caregivers / Maria M. Meyer and Paula Derr, RN,
BSN, CEN, CCRN.—Fourth edition.
  pages cm
  Includes index.
  Previously published as: The comfort of home :
a complete guide for caregivers. 2007.
  ISBN 97809851391-5-5
  ISBN 97809851391-4-8

 1. Home care services--Handbooks, manuals, etc.
2. Caregivers--Handbooks, manuals, etc.   I. Derr, Paula.
II. Title.

RA645.3.M49 2013   362.14
                             QBI13-600181

Text Illustration: Stacey L. Tandberg
Interior Design: Frank Loose
Cover Design: Carlos Maldonado
Page Layout: Lapiz Inc.

Printed in the United States of America.

14 15 16 17 18 /10 9 8 7 6 5 4 3 2 1

About the Authors

Maria Meyer has been a long-time advocate of social causes, beginning with her work as co-founder of the Society for Abused Children of the Children's Home Society of Florida and founding executive director of the Children's Foundation of Greater Miami. In 1993, when her father-in-law suffered a stroke, Maria became aware of the need for better information about how to care for an aging parent, a responsibility shared by millions of Americans. That experience led Maria to found CareTrust Publications and to co-author the award-winning guide, *The Comfort of Home® A Complete Guide for Caregivers*—now in its fourth edition—earning the Benjamin Franklin Award in the health category and *Finalist* in the Book of the Year award by *ForeWord Reviews*. Maria has co-authored a caregiver guide series—including the MS, Stroke, Parkinson, Alzheimer's, Chronic Lung Disease, Chronic Liver Disease and Chronic Heart Failure—editions. She is a keynote speaker and workshop leader on caregiver topics to health care professionals and community groups, as well as, the Northern California *Caregiver Community Action Network* (CCAN) volunteer for the *Caregiver Action Network* (formerly the National Family Caregiver Association). For more than 10 years, Maria has practiced *Taoist Tai Chi®* and is a Beginning Instructor of the Taoist Tai Chi Society of the USA, Inc. Maria and her husband live in San Francisco.

Paula Derr has been employed by the Sisters of Providence Health System for over 37 years. The past seven years she has been working in the Quality Management office as Quality Coordinator. She is author of emergency medical services field guides for emergency medical technicians (EMTs), paramedics, and nurses and has co-authored numerous health care articles. For Paula, home care is a family tradition of long standing. For many years, Paula cared for her mother and grandmother in her home while raising two daughters and maintaining her career in nursing and health care management. Her personal and professional experience adds depth to many chapters of this book. Paula is active in several prominent professional organizations—OrAHQ, NAHQ, ENA,and AACN, —and is an officer on the OrAHQ Board. Paula is a native Oregonian and lives with her husband in Portland.

Our Mission

CareTrust Publications is committed to providing high-quality, user-friendly information to those who face an illness or the responsibilities of caring for friends, family, or clients.

❧

Dedication

Dedicated with loving respect to Marian, Lula, and Ciocia, caregivers of body and spirit. Their loving and selfless spirits inspire me daily. *M.M.M.*

In memory of my mother and grandmother, who lovingly allowed me to care for them in my home. *P.D.*

Dear Caregiver,

This new, fourth edition, has many important and welcome updates—the Affordable Care Act, tax rules, new CPR procedures and an expanded chapter on preventing caregiver burnout. We have no doubt that this fourth edition will be the go-to book for family and para-professional caregivers.

Caring for someone with a chronic or debilitating illness can be deeply satisfying as well as uniquely challenging. Partners, family, and friends can be drawn more closely together when they meet these challenges. Yet, caregiving can also be physically and emotionally exhausting, especially for the person who is the primary caregiver.

Caregiving in The Comfort of Home®: A Complete Guide for Caregivers is a basic but complete guide to answering your questions about caregiving. This guide to in-home care uses current best practices in the areas it covers. It offers practical tips for the activities of daily living as well as the more complicated and stressful situations a caregiver may face. It also includes a wide-ranging list of resources for further reading and study. *Caregiving in The Comfort of Home®* book series offers volumes on specific diseases, such as Alzheimer's. We refer you to those editions for disease-specific conditions.

The *Guide* is divided into three parts:

Part One, Getting Ready, describes how to prepare for the task of caregiving. It shows how to set up a home in a safe and comfortable way for the person whose needs are changing and abilities are declining because of an illness. Perhaps most important, it teaches you how to communicate better with doctors, nurses, aides, pharmacists and insurance companies to get the services you need.

Part Two, Day by Day, takes you through every aspect of daily care. This may be as basic as activities of daily living, such as bathing or helping someone transfer from a chair to a bed, or as daring as traveling abroad with a person whose health is declining.

Part Three, Additional Resources, provides a list of common medical abbreviations to help you understand the terms that many health care-professionals use. There is information about medical specialists who can be part of the health care team and a glossary of terms used to describe and explain symptoms or conditions.

Because a picture is worth a thousand words, we frequently use illustrations throughout the *Guide*. We also include information on organizations and publications that will be invaluable in helping you provide care.

Being a caregiver is not for the timid and fearful. However, having as much knowledge as possible will help you overcome your fears. With this *Guide* in hand, you will understand what help is needed and learn where to find it or how to provide it yourself.

Warm regards,

Maria & Paula

Maria and Paula

Acknowledgments

The procedures described in this *Guide* are based on research and consultation with experts in the fields of nursing, medicine, and design. The authors thank the innumerable professionals and caregivers who have assisted in the development of this book. We are especially grateful to the following reviewers who made comments on sections of the manuscript during its development. We thank them for their significant contributions, without which the quality and comprehensiveness of this Guide would not have been possible. Some sections of this volume are adapted from other editions in *The Comfort of Home®* series. We extend our gratitude to those authors and organizations whose contributions have enhanced this book.

David Abrams
President
Hospice Foundation of America

Judy Alleman, RN, MN
CNS, Gerontology Professor
Mental Health Nursing
Clark College

Mary J. Amdall-Thompson, RN, MS
Program Executive-Professional Services
Oregon Board of Nursing

Julie Barsukoff Kornilkin
Caregiver

Sonya Beebe, RN
Executive Director
Elder Abode, Lincoln City, Oregon

Brad Bowman, MD
CEO, WellMed, Inc.

Beth Boyd-Roberts, PT
Physical Therapy–In-Patient Supervisor

Jon Caswell
Lead Editor, *Stroke Connection Magazine*

Karen Foley, OTR
Director, Regional Rehabilitation Services

Ruth Freeman, CNA
Caregiver

Kay B. Girsberger, RD

Bonnie O. Houston

Rees C. Johnston, JD

Ray Jordan, CPA

Casey C. Kellar
Author, *The Natural Beauty & Bath Book*

Esther King, RN, MN
Professor of Nursing, Clark College

Toni Lonning, MSW, LCSW
Social Worker/Care Manager

Betty McCallum, RN, BSN

Sylvia McSkimming, PhD, RD
Executive Director
Supportive Care of the Dying:
A Coalition for Compassionate Care

To Our Readers

We believe *Caregiving in The Comfort of Home®: A Complete Guide for Caregivers* reflects currently accepted practice in the areas it covers. However, the authors and publisher assume no liability with respect to the accuracy, completeness, or application of information presented here.

Caregiving in The Comfort of Home® is not meant to replace medical care but to add to the medical advice and services you receive from health care professionals. You should seek professional medical advice from a health care provider. This book is only a guide; follow your common sense and good judgment.

Neither the authors nor the publisher are engaged in rendering legal, accounting, or other professional advice. Seek the services of a competent professional if legal, architectural, or other expert assistance is required. The Guide does not represent Americans with Disabilities Act compliance.

Every effort has been made at the time of publication to provide accurate names, addresses, and phone numbers in the resource sections at the ends of chapters. The resources listed are those that benefit readers nationally. For this reason we have not included many local groups that offer valuable assistance. Failure to include an organization does not mean that it does not provide a valuable service. On the other hand, inclusion does not imply an endorsement. The authors and publisher do not warrant or guarantee any of the products described in this book and did not perform any independent analysis of the products described.

Throughout the book, we use "he" and "she" interchangeably when referring to the caregiver and the person being cared for.

ATTENTION NONPROFIT ORGANIZATIONS, CORPORATIONS, AND PROFESSIONAL ORGANIZATIONS: *Caregiving in The Comfort of Home®* is available at special quantity discounts for bulk purchases for gifts, fundraising, or educational training purposes. Special books, book excerpts, or booklets can also be created to fit specific needs. For details, visit www.comfortofhome.com or email resources@comfortofhome.com or call (800) 565-1533.

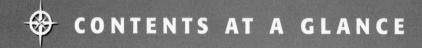

CONTENTS AT A GLANCE

Praise for *The Comfort of Home*® Caregiver Guides

"This is an invaluable addition to bibliographies for the home caregiver. Hospital libraries will want to have a copy on hand for physicians, nurses, social workers, chaplains, and any staff dealing with MS patients and their caregivers. Highly recommended for all public libraries and consumer health collections."
—*Library Journal*

"A well-organized format with critical information and resources at your fingertips . . . educates the reader about the many issues that stand before people living with chronic conditions and provides answers and avenues for getting the best care possible."
—MSWorld, Inc. www.msworld.org

"A masterful job of presenting the multiple aspects of caregiving in a format that is both comprehensive and reader-friendly . . . important focus on physical aspects of giving care."
—Parkinson Report

"Almost any issue or question or need for resolution is most likely spoken of somewhere within the pages of this guide."
—*American Journal of Alzheimer's Disease*

"Physicians, family practitioners and geriatricians, and hospital social workers should be familiar with the book and recommend it to families of the elderly."
—Reviewers Choice, Home Care University

"An excellent guide on caregiving in the home. Home health professionals will find it to be a useful tool in teaching family caregivers."
—Five Star Rating, *Doody's Health Sciences Review Journal*

"Overall a beautifully designed book with very useful, practical information for caregivers."
—Judges from the Benjamin Franklin Awards

"Noteable here are the specifics. Where others focus on psychology alone, this gets down to the nitty gritty."
—*The Midwest Book Review*

"We use *The Comfort of Home*™ for the foundational text in our 40-hour Caregiver training. I believe it is the best on the market."
—Linda Young, Project Manager, College of the Desert

Part One: Getting Ready

Chapter

Is Home Care for You?

Is Home Care for You?

The need to provide care for another person arises for many reasons. Often, the person who needs care does not realize it and family members must step in to help make decisions. One of those decisions involves who the caregiver will be and where care will be provided. The choices can be difficult unless you know what to consider.

When one member of the family becomes disabled or ill, roles within the family often change. A person who took care of the family in the past or was the income provider may become dependent, while another person in the family takes on added, often unfamiliar responsibilities. For a single person, the changes may involve a new dependence on non-family members. Just the word "dependence" can cause unpleasant feelings. Being able to talk openly about fears, anxiety, frustration, and doubts can be very helpful in dealing well with these new facts of life.

Discuss chronic care needs with the person's medical team to learn what treatments, adjustments and other changes may be necessary (see chapter 2). For some people, training to provide medical treatments, advice on coping with the challenges of chronic illness, and some long-range financial planning will be enough. For others, in-home personal assistance is the best option. Sometimes a skilled nursing home or assisted living center is the better choice for everyone involved.

In making the decision for home care, it is important to be realistic about what the person in your care needs, and what you, the caregiver, can provide in terms of time, kinds of care, and financial responsibility. For example, deciding to hire an in-home attendant may be necessary if the primary caregiver works full time. Before this happens, it's important to look at the financial and emotional issues that go along with this decision.

Caregivers need to think about important issues such as independence, privacy, and the financial effect of hiring in-home help. Then the caregiver needs to talk to the person with the illness and others living in the home about these issues. How will the family pay for in-home help and how will it find the right person(s) or agency?

Before a person can be hired, the family needs to look at what kind of care is needed: **medical** *(symptom management, occupational or physical therapies, etc.),* **personal care** *(bathing, dressing, using the bathroom, etc.),* **homemaking** *(shopping, errands, laundry, housecleaning), or* **companionship** *(social outlets, safety issues, etc.).*

Your Support System

Sometimes children take on major household and personal care duties when a parent has disability. Although it is positive for children to take on household jobs and tasks, their needs must be carefully balanced with the amount and level of caregiving they are expected to provide. Children are not equipped to handle the stress of being the main or primary caregiver. They should never be in charge of a parent's medical treatments or daily functions, such as helping with the bathroom.

Family and friends can help. The first step is to let friends and family know that their help is needed and welcomed. Friends often worry that offering help might seem like meddling, especially when things seem to be going well.

Knowing What Level of Care Is Needed

Before you take on the demanding job of home care, decide what level of care you must provide. Do you need to give:

- minimum assistance?

- moderate assistance?

- maximum assistance?

In order to decide what level of care is needed, you must understand the person's condition and needs in the areas of daily care and health. Generally, these needs fall into two broad groups:

Activities of Daily Living (ADLs) such as eating, bathing, dressing, taking medicine, and going to the toilet.

Instrumental Activities of Daily Living (IADLs) are activities that are important to independence, such as cooking, shopping, housekeeping, getting to the doctor, paying bills, and managing money.

Things to look for in deciding the overall level of care needed are the person's

- ability to get from bed to wheelchair without help
- ability to move without help in wheelchair or walker
- ability to manage bladder and bowel
- ability to carry out the basic activities of daily living
- ability to call for help
- degree of sight and hearing impairment
- degree of confusion

Also, consider emotional conditions that might require advanced or special levels of care:

- depression
- a need to be with other people or to have privacy
- homesickness

After giving some thought to the level of care that might be needed and the person's condition, abilities, and emotional state, try to place the person you might care for in one of these categories:

Minimum Assistance—This person is basically independent, can handle most household chores and personal care, and needs help with only one or two activities of daily living.

Moderate Assistance—This person needs help with three or more activities of daily living, such as bathing, cooking, or shopping.

Maximum Assistance—This person is unable to care for himself or herself, requires total assistance, and must be placed in a nursing home if no skilled caregiver is available in the home. Care is often provided by professionals, either in the home through home service agencies or in an adult care homes, assisted living facilities, or nursing homes. At this level, serious problems are a real possibility.

Deciding Whether Home Care Is Possible

When a person has a chronic condition or a terminal illness, daily long-term skilled help with health and personal needs may be in order. Whatever level of care is needed, it can take place in three settings:

- the person's own home

- your home

- residential care facilities, such as an adult care home, assisted living, or a skilled nursing facility

Home Care Considerations

Whether care will take place in your home or in the home of the person who needs care, the following factors must be considered:

- Is there enough room for both the person and items such as a wheelchair, walker, bedside toilet, and lift?

- How accessible is the home if walkers or wheelchairs are used?

- Is a doctor, nurse, or specialist available to supervise care when needed?

- Is there a hospital emergency unit close by?

- Is the home environment safe and supportive, and does it allow for some independence?

- Is money available to hire additional help?

- Is the person in question willing to have a caregiver in the home?

- Can the caregiver manage this role along with other family and personal responsibilities?

Things That Must Be Provided

- Medication

- Meals

- Personal care

- Housecleaning

- Shopping

- Transportation

- Coordinating doctors appointments

- Companionship

- Accessibility (home modification wheelchair ramps, support railings, and changes to the bath and shower stall) (See **Preparing the Home**, p. 113)

Benefits of Home Care

- When a caregiver's spouse or partner is supportive, the experience can strengthen the relationship.

- The relationship between the caregiver and the care receiver can grow stronger.

- A great deal of money can be saved on health care costs.

Why Home Care May Not Be Possible

- Financial reasons (inadequate health insurance to cover the cost of home nursing)

- Family limits (lack of time or money)

- The caregiver's lack of physical and emotional strength

- The person's complex medical condition

- The home's physical layout

- The person's desire to live independently of family

Possible Hazards of Home Care

- Possible lack of freedom for the caregiver.

- Caregiver duties may affect the caregiver's job, career, hobbies, and personal life.

- There may be less time for family members, and the caregiver's family relationships may suffer.

- Children in the home may need to be quieter.

- There may be less time for regular social contacts, religious services, and volunteer work.

- Friends and family may criticize the caregiver's efforts and offer unwelcome advice.

- The caregiver may often be awakened during the night.

- The caregiver may feel unable to control life's events and may suffer from depression, worry, anger, regrets, guilt, and stress.

- Instead of being grateful, the person receiving care may display unpleasant changes in attitude.

- The person receiving care may react to constant daily irritations by lashing out at the caregiver.

- The caregiver may begin to fear the time when he or she may be dependent on someone for care.

- The caregiver may feel obliged to spend personal funds on caregiving.

- The caregiver may become physically ill and emotionally drained.

Outside Help

One of the biggest pitfalls in caregiving is trying to do it all yourself. But other help is available and should be called on whenever possible. That help includes:

- Support groups

- Day care and respite care, which provide relief for the caregiver

- Organizations providing respite care

- Pastoral or other counseling services

- Agency or parish nurses

- Medical services provided by professionals, such as nurses and therapists

- Personal services for the person in your care, such as grooming or dressing, provided by home health aides

- Community home health services on a fee basis, such as Professional Geriatric Managers or Visiting Nurse Associations (see *Getting In-Home Help*, p. 49)

Checklist **The Caregiver**

The ideal caregiver is—

✓ *emotionally and physically capable of handling the work*

✓ *able to share duties and responsibilities with other willing family members*

✓ *able to plan solutions and solve problems instead of withdrawing under stress*

✓ *able to speak in a simple and clear way*

✓ *comfortable giving and receiving help*

✓ *trained for the level of care required*

✓ *able to handle unpleasant tasks such as changing diapers, bathing, or treating bed sores*

✓ *in good health and has energy, skill, and the ability to adapt*

✓ *able to cope with anger and frustration*

✓ *able to afford respite (non-caregiving time) care when necessary*

✓ *able to speak to and understand the care receiver*

✓ *able to make this person feel useful and needed*

✓ *valued by other family members*

✓ *able to adjust to the future needs and wishes of the person in care*

✓ *aware of other care options and willing to explore them*

If you have most of these traits, you may be a good candidate to provide home care. However, consider the list called "Possible Hazards of Home Care" on page 9 and be honest with yourself about your ability to cope.

Supportive Housing and Care Options

If you believe that home care is not practical for you, many other options exist. Good programs foster independence, dignity, privacy, a very high level of functioning, and connections with the community. However, people who have lived independently all their lives may not be suited to live in groups, and those who are mentally alert or are younger may be very unhappy living with people who suffer from dementia.

Keep the above factors in mind when you check out the following:

- **Independent Living Options**—apartment buildings, condos, retirement communities, and single-family homes

- **Semi-independent Living Options**—for those with lower incomes, these places offer the same benefits as independent living but also include meal service and housekeeping as part of the monthly fee, provide help with personal care, keep track of health and medications, and provide special diets. These options are frequently offered in assisted living facilities and group homes sometimes at an additional cost.

- **Skilled Care Facilities**—nursing homes

NOTE States use different names for care facilities. The services can also vary, so it is important to check with the facility and each state's licensing agency to confirm exactly which services are offered. For example, in Wyoming, assisted living allows people who are unrelated to share a room. In some other places, living spaces are not shared, except by personal choice.

A Closer Look at the Options

House Sharing—for people who are fully independent

- Two or more unrelated people live together, each with a private bedroom.

- All living areas are shared.

- Chores and expenses are shared.

- Personal-assistant services may be shared.

Group Homes or Adult Homes—homes in residential neighborhoods for people whose needs vary, from assistance with individual services to dependent residents with increased nursing services

- Care is given to small groups of people in the primary caregiver's home or with a live-in resident manager/caregiver.

- The home is privately run and provides private or shared rooms with meals, housekeeping, personal care (such as bathing and dressing), keeping track of medication, safety supervision, and some transportation.

- Rates vary according to individual care needs, and Medicaid funding is often available for repayment to those who qualify.

- Staff are qualified and facilities are licensed according to the level of services offered, which can include housekeeping, laundry, personal care assistance, bathing, dressing, grooming, and management of medication and other medical needs, such as injections or inability to control bladder and bowel.

NOTE Some states do not license, inspect, or keep watch over adult care homes. Before selecting one, call your local Area Agency on Aging or the state or county Department of Health and Human Services to see if any complaints have been filed against the home you are considering.

Assisted Living Facilities—for moderate assistance to those who are frail and usually require assistance with activities of daily living

• Each person lives in his or her own apartment.

• An emergency staff is available 24 hours a day.

• Monthly charges are based on the level of service needed.

• Activities such as games, hobbies, crafts, and music are offered.

• Meals, housekeeping, medication management, and nursing assessment are provided.

• Transportation and access to medical services can be arranged.

NOTE There is no national control over these facilities, but there is state licensing and regulation. For information on a specific facility, call the ombudsman in your state or the state agency that licenses the facility. (An ombudsman is someone who investigates complaints made by individuals.)

Continuing Care Retirement Communities—for people who want a range of services from independent living to nursing home care

• These facilities provide a lifetime contract for care.

• They provide or offer meals and can handle special diets.

- They offer housekeeping, scheduled transportation, emergency help, personal care, and activities for fun and learning.

- Many retirement communities require entrance fees that can vary quite a bit.

- They also have monthly fees ranging from several hundred to several thousand dollars.

- Some provide home health care and nursing home care without extra fees.

- Some charge extra for nursing unit residents.

Skilled nursing or convalescent Homes—for people who require continuous and ongoing nursing assistance or monitoring

Nursing homes typically offer three levels of care:

- **Custodial**—minimal nursing, but help with hygiene, meals, dressing, etc.

- **Intermediate**—help for those who cannot live alone but do not need 24-hour skilled nursing care

- **Skilled Nursing**—intensive 24-hour skilled nursing care

Hospice care is available in most settings as a covered benefit under Medicare. It is also covered for those who receive Medicaid in states that offer hospice coverage under their Medicaid program.

Tip

Medicaid is a joint federal and state program, and the states have some flexibility in setting the benefits they will offer and the eligibility criteria for those benefits.

Financing Options

The choice of the right housing option may depend on financing available:

- **Personal Resources** are the most common way to pay.

- **Private Insurance** is helpful, but some policies limit the length and type of benefits and have waiting periods or other limits.

- **Medicare** is for those 65 and older or for people who have been declared disabled by the Social Security Administration. Medicare partially pays for up to 100 days in a skilled nursing care facility after a qualifying related hospitalization of more than three days in a row (not including the day the person leaves the hospital). The financing of hospice care is a separate benefit under Medicare.

- **Medicaid** partially pays for services, including assisted living services in some states, to those who are aged, blind, or have disabilities and have limited financial resources. It is also a major payer for nursing home care.

> **Tip**
>
> In a private pay facility, if your money runs out, you can't stay unless they take public benefits such as Medicaid. Remember, before choosing a facility, make sure that in addition to private pay they also accept public benefits such as Social Security or Medicaid.

- **Medigap** policies cover gaps in coverage and may be in place to pay Medicare coinsurance. (📖 See *Financial Management,* p. 73)

Checklist **Review Before Deciding on a Facility**

✓ Is a trial period allowed to be sure a person is happy with the facility?

✓ Will the facility refund deposits or entrance fees if the resident dies, chooses to leave, or is asked to leave?

✓ Can a resident choose his or her own apartment? Can personal furniture be used?

✓ Are there younger residents at the facility?

✓ If the person must be away for a short time (even for a hospital stay), will the same apartment be available when he or she returns? Is there a reduced rate during long absences?

✓ If the person marries, can the couple live in the same apartment?

✓ Can the staff handle special diets? Are meal menus posted?

✓ Is transportation provided?

✓ How many people are on staff, and how much training have they had?

✓ How often and for what reasons can staff enter the apartment?

✓ Can the resident see his or her own doctor? Who gives out the medications?

✓ Is physical therapy available within the facility?

✓ Is the facility licensed to deal with a resident whose health gets worse or must the person leave if, for example, he or she can no longer walk or begins arguing or fighting with others?

✓ How are decisions made when a person must be moved to another part of the facility?

✓ Is there a 30-day-notice provision for ending the agreement?

✓ Does the facility take Medicare?

✓ Will the facility let a resident "spend down" his or her assets and go on Medicaid?

Points to Review Before Signing a Contract or Lease

Although it is hard to know what problems may arise in a care setting, it is extremely important to take the following steps before signing any legal papers:

- Find out who owns the facility and review the owner's financial status.

- Ask for a copy of the contract before signing and review it with an attorney, financial advisor, or a trusted family member.

- Do not rely on spoken promises. Make sure the contract is geared to the resident's needs.

- Read the state inspection report on the facility.

- Read all the rules and policies of the facility that are not in the contract.

- Ask to see the facility's license.

If you have access to a computer or smartphone, Google the facility to see what others have said about it.

Things You Should Know About Facilities

Residents' Rights

General Rights—Residents maintain all their rights guaranteed under the U.S. Constitution, including the right to vote. In addition, they can receive visitors, voice their concerns, form resident councils, and enjoy informed consent, privacy, and freedom of choice.

Privacy—In some cases, a resident may have a roommate. However, residents' rooms are considered private, and staff must knock before entering. Also, residents can have private visits with spouses.

Restraints—Only the resident's doctor may order a restraint as part of a care plan, and the doctor must state the specific restraint's use and period of use. (Use of restraints is strongly discouraged, although not prohibited.)

Lifestyle Choices—Residents do not have as many choices as they would have at home regarding meal times, menu choices, and times for sleep. However, most facilities try to satisfy residents' needs as much as possible.

Ability to Effect Change—Issues can be brought up to the resident council or the long-term care ombudsman.

Freedom to Leave—If a person with legal capacity chooses to enter a facility, then she has the right to leave at any time regardless of concerns or what the family thinks after giving at least 30 days' written notice to the facility.

 The following describes general guidelines regarding a resident's rights. To obtain specific rules for a particular state, contact the state agency responsible for licensing the facility.

The Resident's Rights When Leaving a Facility

Depending on the admission agreement, a resident must be given 30 days written notice before being moved. If there is a medical emergency, no written notice is required. Generally, a resident may be moved from a facility for the following reasons:

- The person wants to be moved.

- The person must be moved for his or her own good.

- The person must be moved for the good of other residents.

- The facility is not being paid. (However, someone who runs out of money may not be moved if Medicaid will pay and they are living at a Medicaid facility.)

- The person came into the facility for special care and that care is completed.

- The facility is being closed.

If the person does not want to leave the facility, IMMEDIATELY contact the state agency responsible for licensing the facility and/or Medicaid certification.

If you have questions, call the following:

- the Center for Medicare-Medicaid Services (CMS)

- the local Aging and Disabled Services Division of the Department of Health and Human Resources

- the long-term care ombudsman

- the Federal Health Care Financing Administration

- the local Area Agency on Aging

- a nonprofit agency focused on elder law or a legal hot line

What Family Members and Friends Should Do

- Visit whenever possible.

- Send cards or letters between visits.

- Bring small gifts and treats.

- If allowed, walk around with the person when visiting to provide exercise.

- Listen to the resident's complaints.

- Build a good relationship with the staff.

- Plan off-site outings if appropriate.

*R*ESOURCES ➤

Caring.com
www.Caring.com
The leading online destination for family caregivers seeking information, support, in-home care and senior living options. Provides free, personalized help finding the right care for your loved one. Provides a directory to find senior living options in every state.

AARP
601 E Street, NW
Washington, DC 20049
1-888-OUR-AARP (1-888-687-2277) (voice)
(877) 434-7598 (tty)
member@aarp.org
www.aarp.org
Web site provides information, articles, blogs on caregiving and other aging issues.

National Council on Independent Living
1710 Rhode Island Avenue NW, Fifth Floor
Washington, DC 20036
(877) 525-3400 (voice)
(202) 207-0340 (tty)
ncil@ncil.org
www.ncil.org
Refers callers to their state's independent-living centers. Offers publications and advice related to disability issues. Advocates for adult disabled and policy changes.

Family Caregiver Alliance, National Center on Caregiving
785 Market Street, Suite 750
(415) 434-3388
For 50-state resources, the National Center can be reached
9:00 A.M. to 5:00 P.M. (PT) M-F
(800) 445-8106
http://www.caregiver.org/

Assisted Living Facilities and Nursing Homes

Leading Edge
2519 Connecticut Avenue, NW
Washington, DC 20008
(202) 783-2242 (voice)
(202) 783-2255 (fax)
info@leadingage.org
www.leadingage.org
Provides information on not-for-profit nursing homes, senior housing facilities, assisted living, and community services.

American Health Care Association/National Center for Assisted Living
1201 L Street, NW
Washington, DC 20005
(202) 842-4444
http://www.ahcancal.org/
Provides consumer information on services, financing, public policy, nursing facilities, assisted living, and subacute care. Represents more than 11,000 providers of assisted living, nursing care, and subacute care.

Assisted Living Federation of America
1650 King Street, Suite 602
Alexandria, VA 22314
(703) 894-1805
www.alfa.org
Offers referrals to local facilities listed by state. Provides several downloadable guides, checklists, and toolkits.

The **Center for Medicare and Medicaid Services** has detailed information about the past performance of every Medicare- and Medicaid-certified nursing home in the country. For more information, go to www.medicare.gov, click on Search Tools at the top of the page, and then click on Compare Nursing Homes in Your Area. For a list of **Medicare-certified nursing homes**, call the local office or department on aging.

Housing and Urban Development (HUD)
For homeowner help or those seeking affordable housing, HUD has a state-by-state guide, see
http://portal.hud.gov/hudportal/HUD

Respite Services

ARCH National Respite Locator Service
800 Eastowne Drive, Suite 105
Chapel Hill, NC 27514-2204
(919) 490-5577
mmathers@chtop.org
www.respitelocator.org
Provides caregivers with contact information on respite services in their area.

Family Care Navigator
Family Caregiver Alliance
www.caregiver.org
Lists state-by-state and national resources. Search "Family Care Navigator".

Eldercare Locator
National Association of Area Agencies on Aging
1730 Rhode Island Avenue, NW, Suite 1200
Washington, DC 20036
(800) 677-1116
www.eldercare.gov
www.n4a.org
Supplies information about many eldercare issues, including respite care. Provides referrals to local respite programs and local Area Agency on Aging.

If you don't have access to the Internet, ask your local library or senior center to help you locate a Web site.

For a list of **Medicare Certified Nursing Homes,** call the local Office on Aging.

Using the Health Care Team Effectively

Using the Health Care Team Effectively

When you care for someone in the home, you must also manage that person's health care. This means choosing a good medical team, keeping costs down, arranging for medical appointments, and getting the best, least expensive medicines. It also means knowing what the insurance rules are and, most importantly, being an advocate (a supporter) for the person in your care.

Doctors and nurses can focus on physical diagnosis and may ignore the emotional aspects of care. Sometimes they have little time to consider the spiritual aspects of healing. Although you should consult with professionals about the levels of therapy and support needed for the person in your care, you do not have to accept what they suggest or order. Keep asking questions until you completely understand the diagnosis (what is wrong), treatment, and prognosis (likely outcome).

Choosing a Doctor

Call your local medical or dental society for the names of doctors who specialize in the field in which you seek care. Think about using doctors who are allied with medical schools. They tend to have the most up-to-date information, especially about complicated illnesses.

- Always make sure the doctor is board certified in his or her specialty.

- If the person in your care is enrolled in an HMO, ask if the doctor is planning to change HMOs anytime soon.

- You can contact more than one doctor (for a second opinion). If you are enrolled in Medicare Supplementary Medical Insurance (Part B), Medicare will pay for a second opinion in the same way it pays for other services. After Part B of the deductible has been met, Medicare pays 80 percent of the Medicare-approved amount for a second opinion and will provide the same coverage for a third opinion.

Tip

You can change doctors anytime you feel uncomfortable about the care provided.

Nurse Practitioners

Seek out a medical practice that incorporates the services of a nurse practitioner or physician assistant. These mid-level practitioners provide health screening, perform physical examinations, order laboratory tests, and prescribe specific medications authorized by the physician. Nurse practitioners also educate patients about staying healthy. Often they are the best-equipped health professionals to educate patients and caregivers about the common problems of chronic illness. Mid-level health care providers usually spend more time with patients and caregivers than the supervising medical specialists in a busy practice.

How to Share in Medical Decisions

In the end, medical decision-making is in the hands of the person receiving care, the doctor, and the caregiver. Learn to take an active role and become an advocate for yourself and for the person in your care. It has been said that a patient is the senior partner in the patient–doctor relationship.

Long-Range Considerations

- Find out how the person in your care feels about treatments that prolong life. Respect these views.

- Help the person receiving care to set up an advance directive and power of attorney for health care. (📖 See *Planning for End-of-Life Care*, p. 107)

- Share decisions with the doctor and the care receiver and take responsibility for the treatment and its outcomes.

The Doctor–Patient–Caregiver Relationship

- Be aware that doctors must see more patients per day than they once did.

- Be aware that some doctors may have financial reasons for doing too much or too little for those in their care. Specialists are often the only ones with the training needed to treat a serious or chronic condition, so the doctor may refer the care receiver to a specialist.

- If the relationship with the doctor becomes unfriendly, find a new doctor.

- Respect the doctor's time (you may need to have more than one visit to cover all issues).

- If Medicare is the payer, ask if the doctor accepts Medicare assignment. If not, the difference may have to be paid out of pocket.

Preparing for a Visit to the Doctor

- Be prepared to briefly explain the care receiver's and the family's medical history.

- Take a list of questions in order of importance.

- Prepare a list of any symptoms the person you care for is experiencing.

- Be prepared to ask for written information on the medical situation so you can better understand what the doctor is saying, or bring a small tape recorder.

- You can call the hospital's library or health resource center for help in looking up any questions the doctor does not answer.

 Be sure shots for tetanus, flu, and pneumonia are up-to-date. For those on Medicare, flu and pneumonia shots may be covered.

At the Doctor's Office

- Tell the doctor what you hope and expect from the visit and any recommended treatment.

- If the doctor tells you to do something you know you can't do, such as give medication in the middle of the night, ask if there is another treatment and explain why.

- Insist on talking about the level of care that you believe is appropriate and that agrees with the care receiver's wishes.

- Ask about other options for tests, medications, and surgery.

- Ask why tests or treatments are needed and what the risks are.

- Consider all options, including the pros and cons of "watchful waiting."

- Trust your common sense and if you have doubts, get a second opinion.

Checklist **Changes to Report to the Doctor**

Contact the doctor right away if the following changes occur. Fever may be caused by an infection and should always be reported:

Ability to Move

✓ *falls, even if there is no pain*

✓ *leg pain when walking*

✓ *painful or limited movement (color of skin over painful areas should be reported)*

✓ *inability to move*

Diet

✓ *extreme thirst*

✓ *lack of thirst*

✓ *weight loss for no reason*

✓ *loss of appetite*

✓ *pain before or after eating*

✓ *difficulty chewing or swallowing*

✓ *pain in the gums or teeth*

✓ *frequent gum infections*

Behavior

✓ *unusual tiredness or sleepiness*

✓ *unusual actions (arguing, fighting, anger, or withdrawal)*

✓ *seeing or hearing things that aren't there (hallucinations)*

✓ *anxiety*

✓ *increased confusion*

✓ *depression*

✓ *inappropriate or unusual emotions*

✓ *loss of memory and forgetfulness*

Bowel/Bladder

✓ *bowel movements of an odd color, texture, or amount*

✓ *feeling faint during bowel movements*

✓ *vaginal discharge (report color, odor, amount)*

✓ *draining sores or pain in the penis area*

✓ *pain when going to the bathroom (unusual color, amount, or odor)*

✓ *having to go to the bathroom frequently*

✓ *frequent bladder infections*

✓ *blood in the urine*

✓ *pain in the kidney area*

Skin

- ✓ changes in the color of lips, nails, fingers, and toes
- ✓ odd skin (color, temperature, texture, bruises)
- ✓ unusual appearance of surgery incisions
- ✓ sudden skin rashes (bumps, itching)
- ✓ pressure sores (bedsores)

Bones, Muscles, and Joints

- ✓ swelling in the arms and legs or around the eyes
- ✓ twitching or movement that cannot be controlled
- ✓ tingling or numbness in hands, feet, and other parts of the body
- ✓ warm, tender joints
- ✓ redness in the joints
- ✓ unusual position of arms, legs, fingers, or toes

Chest

- ✓ chest pain
- ✓ rapid pulse

- ✓ problems with breasts (report lumps, discharge, soreness, or draining)
- ✓ painful breathing (wheezing, shortness of breath)
- ✓ unusual cough
- ✓ unusual saliva or mucus (report color and consistency)

Abdomen

- ✓ stomach pain
- ✓ vomiting

Head

- ✓ dizziness
- ✓ headaches
- ✓ ear pain, discharge, or change in hearing
- ✓ eye pain, discharge, redness, blurry vision, or being bothered by light
- ✓ mouth sores
- ✓ nose pain (bleeding, bad odor to mucus)

KEEP ASKING QUESTIONS UNTIL YOU ARE SATISFIED. Doctors and other health care professionals have medical know-how, but only you can explain symptoms. Report exactly, in as few words as possible, any unusual symptoms, changes in condition, and complaints the person has.

If the Person in Your Care Is Near Death

- Some doctors may not be trained to talk about death and the dying process with their patients, so be prepared to begin the conversation. If you do your search on current death and dying information, you could enlighten your doctor about your request.

- If the person in your care wants to die at home, say this clearly to the doctor.

- Be sure that any directives for health care for the person are available and prominently displayed.

Questions to Ask Before Agreeing to Tests, Medications, and Surgery

Before you begin discussing medical treatment with the doctor, explain that the person in your care does not want any unnecessary tests or treatments. Then ask these questions:

- Why is this test needed?

- How long will it take? How soon will the results be in?

 If your doctor recommends a procedure and the HMO refuses to cover it, see *Appealing an HMO Decision*, page 86.

- Is the test accurate?

- Is it painful?

- Are there risks with the treatment? Do the benefits outweigh the risks?

- How often will side effects occur, and how long will they last?

- Are X-rays really needed?

- Will the doctor review the test report and explain it in detail?

- May a copy of the report be taken home? (If you have questions, ask to talk to the specialist who made the report.)

- If a test is positive, what course of action should be taken?

- Is the condition going to worsen slowly or rapidly?

- What could happen if the person did not have the test?

- How much does the test cost, and is there a less costly one?

Questions to Ask the Doctor About Medications

Medications can be costly, confusing to use, and have unwanted side effects. Be sure to ask questions when medicines are prescribed and prescriptions are filled.

- Give the doctor a list of all medications and dosages that the person in your care is now taking, including eye drops, vitamins, and herbal remedies.

- Tell the doctor of any other treatments being used. Sometimes using two or more treatments may be fatal or may keep the new treatment from working.

- Tell the doctor of any allergies or if there are certain foods the person cannot eat (food allergies).

- Understand why each medication is needed and how much it will help the person's condition.

- Ask if pain can be relieved almost completely, and then ask for the medicine that works best.

- Ask how long it takes for the drug to work.

- Find out its side effects.

- Ask if the drug could react with other drugs and what you should do if there are side effects.

- Find out if a change in diet, exercise, reducing stress, or other things can be done.

- If more than one medicine is needed, ask the doctor if they can be taken at the same times each day. If a drug must be taken at a difficult time (for instance, in the middle of the night), ask about another choice.

- Try to find the lowest cost drug. Ask if a generic (non-brand name) drug or another brand in the same drug class is available at a lower cost.

- Be sure that the generic drug will not have a poor effect on the person's condition.

- Ask if a lower dose can be prescribed without bad effects.

- To keep costs down, ask if a higher dose can be safely prescribed and the pill cut in half.

- Ask if you can buy a one-week supply of a new medication to see if the person can handle any possible side effects. Or ask if the physician has free samples to try.

Check out using an iPad or smartphone for using health care apps for caregiving. Visit www.apple.com/itunes and search "medication reminders".

Tip

BUYING MEDICATIONS
Buying medications through mail order is often the cheapest way to buy, but there are other options to save money. Ask if the insurance company has a mail-order program (see *Resources,* page 46).

Questions to Ask the Pharmacist

Some prescription drugs are not covered by health insurance, so shop around for the drug store with the lowest prices and then stay with it. The pharmacist will come to know the care receiver's condition and can advise you about problems that might come up. Managed care plans are permitted to change doctor's orders by giving you a similar version that is cheaper. Do not try cutting drug costs without talking to you doctor about it first.

- Find out the highest allowable charge for a particular drug.

- Ask what over-the-counter drugs the pharmacist suggests for the person's condition (it may be necessary to take more of the drug if it is over-the-counter).

- Ask if the insurance company will pay for the drug the doctor prescribed.

- Ask if the doctor will be called to approve the switch to another drug.

- Find out what generic drug can be used instead of the brand-name drug.

- Ask if the generic drug can cause side effects and when the doctor should be called about them.

- Ask if using more than one drug can cause unsafe drug interactions.

- Ask if the pharmacy's computer will alert the pharmacist about drug interactions or side effects before the prescription is filled.

- Find out the risks of not taking the medicine.

- Find out the risks of not finishing the prescription.

- If you are caring for someone who will be taking several medications on his or her own, find a drug store that has easy-to-use packaging.

- Ask if the medicine can be put in a large, easy-to-open container with a label in large print.

- Ask if an overdose of the medicine is dangerous.

- Ask if the person can drink alcohol or smoke while taking the medication.

- Ask if the medicine must be taken with a meal, with water or milk, etc.

- When the person needs many expensive drugs, find out if you can get a discount or work out a payment plan.

Tip **MEDICAL ALERT**

An elderly person who is mobile may want to wear a medical alert bracelet or carry a card that lists the medications she is currently taking. The medical alert should carry a contact person's phone number.

Questions to Ask About Surgery

Surgery is a serious step. Ask as many questions as you need before deciding to go ahead.

- Why does the person need the surgery?

- Will the surgery stop the problem or merely slow it down?

- What are the other choices?

- Can it be done on an outpatient basis?

- What will happen if surgery is not done?

- Where will the surgery be done? When?

- Is there a less expensive hospital?

Weigh the age of the patient with the risks and hopeful outcomes:

- Will the surgeon you spoke to do the surgery, or will it be assigned to another doctor? (When going into surgery, put the surgeon's name on the release form to ensure that the named surgeon is the one who does the operation.)

- How many surgeries of this type has the doctor performed? (Generally, the more times the surgeon has performed an operation, the higher the success rate will be.)

- What is the doctor's success rate with this type of surgery?

- What are the anesthesiologist's qualifications?

- What can go wrong?

- How much will the surgery cost, and is it covered by insurance?

- What other specialists can I ask for a second opinion? (Medicaid and Medicare usually pay for second opinions. Doctors expect people to get a second opinion when surgery is needed, and they should help you get one.)

Tip

MEDICAL RECORDS

When seeking a second opinion, to save costs, have all medical records and tests sent to the second doctor. Also, if possible, bring the important ones with you. Even the experts can disagree about the best treatment. The final decision is yours. If time is critical, request medical information be sent electronically.

Alternative Treatments

A healthy lifestyle is encouraged by most medical providers. Use caution if you decide to try a different kind of treatment (known as complementary or alternative treatment). Look before you leap, and follow these commonsense guidelines:

- Be on guard against anyone who says to stop seeing a conventional (regular) doctor or to stop taking prescribed medicine.

- Look into the background of any treatment provider.

- Discuss the alternative or complementary therapy with your doctor.

- Figure out the costs of the treatments.

- Do not abandon conventional therapy.

- Keep a written account of the experience.

Mental Health Treatment

Strong emotions are a normal part of long-term illness. Counseling and support groups are a very helpful way of dealing with these feelings.

- For one who is depressed and needs therapy, ask the primary care doctor to give you the name of a therapist.

- Be aware that many people are embarrassed about mental health problems and may not want to seek care.

- For help determining a person's capacity to make legal decisions, arrange for a neurological evaluation. If the care receiver is elderly, then you may wish to seek out a neurologist with a specialization in geriatrics.

(See **Depression**, p. 255)

Dental Care

Dental care is important for overall wellness. For low-cost dental programs, check with university dental schools or the local Area Agency on Aging.

- Tell the dentist all the medications the person is taking before starting dental treatment.

- Try to go to a dentist who is familiar with the person's disease.

- Find out how many visits will be needed each year.

- Ask if the office and dental chair are accessible, if that is needed.

- Ask about low-cost options to the treatment the dentist suggests.

- Ask if X-rays are really necessary.

- Find out the cost of dentures, but don't trust prices that seem too good to be true. Cheap dentures may not fit correctly.

- When seeking another opinion, have all medical records and tests sent to the second dentist.

Vision Care

Regular eye exams every two years by a specialist in eye disease (ophthalmologist) or someone who examines the eyes (optometrist) are necessary, especially after age 50. These exams can also spot or detect other serious diseases such as diabetes. Finding and treating disease early can prevent serious diseases from getting worse and leading to blindness.

- Tell the doctor of any medicines the person is taking.

- Tell the doctor if there is a family history of glaucoma.

- Get a yearly eye exam for a person with diabetes.

- Contact your state's Commission for the Blind for information on self-help organizations for those with low vision.

- Ask for help in finding products ("talking" watches, etc.) and aids that will help the person adjust to low vision.

- Seek out radio stations that have programs of newspaper readings.

 NOTE Danger signs to watch for are changes in the color or size of an object when one eye is covered or when straight poles appear bent or wavy. See an ophthalmologist (eye doctor) without delay.

How to Watch Out for Someone's Best Interests in the Hospital

A person in the hospital is at greater risk than others, so be ready to keep tabs on treatments, ask questions, and act as an advocate.

- If the Patients' Bill of Rights is not posted in a place where it can be seen, ask for a copy.

- Only consent to treatments that have been thoroughly explained.

- If something is not being done, and you think it should be, ask why.

- Be friendly and show respect to hospital staff. They will probably respond better to you and to the person in your care. Bad feelings between family members and staff may cause the staff to avoid the person.

- Assist with the person's grooming and care.

- Speak up if you notice doctors or nurses examining anyone without first washing their hands.

- Check all bills, and ask questions about charges not clear to you.

Where available, use hospital-grade hand sanitizer to avoid disease-causing germs. It will protect you against germs that regular hand sanitizer will not.

When You Doubt the Time Is Right for Discharge

According to federal law, a hospital must release patients in a *reasonable manner of safety* or else must keep them in the hospital. Letting a patient leave the hospital is not wise if the person has constant fever, open wounds, drainage; requires injections; has infection or pain that cannot be controlled; is confused or disoriented (no sense of time or place); or is unable to take food or liquids by mouth. However, in some cases, it may be better for the person to be released because the noise and risk of catching other diseases may make it more difficult to recover. If you plan to appeal a discharge, understand the rules of Medicare, Medicaid, the HMO, or the person's insurance plan.

Always request a discharge plan with clear instructions in writing because this is your road map of care.

- State your doubts in a simple letter to the hospital's director or the health plan's medical director. (Rules vary from state to state.)

- Meet with the hospital's discharge planner, usually a social worker.

- Ask if the hospital is following the usual policy for the condition.

- Explain any special reasons that make you think it is unwise to discharge the person.

- Ask if the hospital rules can be changed to cover this special case.

- Remember that anyone has the right to appeal a discharge.

- Get your doctor's help in the appeal, but understand that he or she may have different reasons for wanting to discharge the person.

- Request mediation with the care team if a hospital insists on a discharge you disagree with or contact the patient care advocate on staff at most hospitals.

- Beware of hospital's "dumping" patients home to caregivers prematurely in their recovery.

 Hospitals cannot discharge a patient without a plan in place for his or her ongoing care.

Case Management

Case management is an important resource for families living with chronic illness. It is easy to become stressed with the demands of the disease and with the red tape of the health care and social services network. Case managers need to have a basic understanding of the special needs of persons with chronic illness.

Checklist **Coming Home from the Hospital**

✓ Assess the person's condition and needs.

✓ Understand the diagnosis (what is wrong) and prognosis (what will happen).

✓ Become part of the health care team (doctor, nurse, therapists) so you can learn how to provide care.

✓ Get complete written instructions from the doctor. If there is anything you don't understand, ASK QUESTIONS.

✓ Arrange follow-up care from the doctor.

✓ Develop a plan of care with the doctor. (📖 See **Setting Up a Plan of Care,** p. 107)

✓ Meet with the hospital's social worker or discharge planner to determine home care benefits.

✓ Understand in-home assistance options. (See **Getting In-Home Help,** p. 49)

✓ Arrange for in-home help.

✓ Arrange physical, occupational, and speech therapy as needed.

✓ Find out if medicine is provided by the hospital to take home. If not, you will have to have prescriptions filled before you take the person home.

✓ Prepare the home. (📖 See **Preparing the Home,** p. 113)

✓ Buy needed supplies; rent, borrow, or buy equipment such as wheelchairs, crutches, and walkers.

✓ Take home all personal items.

✓ Check with the hospital cashier for discharge payment requirements.

✓ Arrange transportation (an ambulance or van if your car will not do).

Tip Be aware that there may be additional high costs associated with arranged transportation.

> **NOTE** Do not hesitate to call the hospital staff member (ombudsman) who is responsible for patients' rights.

Case management skills are very helpful to families when there is a change in the person's physical state or in awareness and understanding. Should this happen, a case manager can take another look at the person's needs and at community supports. This may be necessary in the following instances:

- When the person loses the ability to process information and help is needed to identify issues and provide follow-up with a course of action

- When there is a change in the caregiver situation or support network that can easily become a crisis for the family as a whole

- When there are fewer financial resources and the family is no longer able to pay for the resources they need

- When safety issues arise that can put the ill person at greater risk

These issues and others require that case management continue as a long-term resource so that the case manager can step in when needed to provide more support.

To learn more about private pay case management or find a case manager in your area, contact:

- **National Association of Professional Geriatric Care Managers**
  3275 West Ina Road, Suite 130
  Tucson, AZ 85741-2198
  (520) 881-8008 (voice)
  (520) 325-7925 (fax)
  http://www.caremanager.org/

- Your local Visiting Nurse Association

- Area Office on Aging

- Hospital discharge planners

If the person in your care has lower income, contact your *county* **Health and Human Services Division** or contact the **U.S. Department of Health and Human Services** at: http://www.hhs.gov/

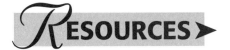 **ESOURCES** ➤

For free or low-cost resources, contact local consumer health resource and information centers (check the local hospital system or phone book) and local health agencies or associations (American Heart Association, American Diabetes Association, National Multiple Sclerosis Society, and others).

WebMD
http://www.webmd.com/

Go Ask Alice!
www.goaskalice.columbia.edu/
Provides helpful information and lets you post health-related questions.

University of Washington
www.uwmedicine.org
Empowering people to live healthier lives around the globe through exceptional patient care, research, and education.

Information About Eyesight

Lighthouse International
111 E. 59th Street
New York, NY 10022
(800) 829-0500
www.lighthouse.org

Lions Club International
300 W. 22nd Street
Oak Brook, IL 60523
(630) 571-5466
http://www.lionsclubs.org/EN/index.php

National Federation of the Blind
200 East Wells Street (at Jernigan Place)
Baltimore, MD 21230
(410) 659-9314
www.nfb.org

Medications

Together Rx Access™ Card
A joint program by drug companies offering a free Prescription Savings Card for individuals and families who meet all four of the following requirements:

❏ *Not eligible for Medicare*

❏ *Household income equal to or less than:*

—*$45,000 for a single person*
—*$60,000 for a family of two*
—*$75,000 for a family of three*
—*$90,000 for a family of four*
—*$105,000 for a family of five*

❏ *Legal resident of the U.S. or Puerto Rico*

Call (800) 444-4106 to start saving on your prescriptions. For the most current list of medicines and products, visit www.TogetherRxAccess.com

NeedyMeds

*The NeedyMeds Drug Discount Card
saves you up to 80% or more off
the cost of:*

❏ *Prescription Medicines*

❏ *Over-the-Counter Drugs*

❏ *Pet Prescription Drugs*

Click on the card to learn more
and get your own card.
http://www.needymeds.org/

Rx Assist

Patient assistance programs are run by pharmaceutical companies to provide free medications to people who cannot afford to buy their medicine. RxAssist offers a comprehensive database of these patient assistance programs, as well as practical tools, news, and articles so that health care professionals and patients can find the information they need all in one place.
http://www.rxassist.org/

WatchMinder

*Vibrating wristwatches, program alerts and messages,
Medication reminders, everyday life and wellness, behavior
modification and self-monitoring, AD/HD, LD, and autism*
http://watchminder.com/

e-Pill

(800) 549-0095
www.epill.com
List of medication reminders.

Patient Advocate Foundation (PAF)
421 Butler Farm Road
Hampton, VA 23666
(800) 532-5274 (voice)
(757) 873-8999 (fax)
www.patientadvocate.org
Resources on insurance and health care access problem and disease-specific information.

NAMI
National Alliance on Mental Illness
The **Information Help-Line** *is an information and referral service that can be reached by calling* **(800) 950-NAMI (6264)**, *Monday through Friday, 10 a.m.–6 p.m., EST or by email at info@nami.org*
http://www.nami.org/

Publication

A Family Caregiver's Guide to Hospital Discharge Planning, a publication of the National Alliance for Caregiving and the United Hospital Fund of New York.
Available at www.caregiving.org

If you don't have access to the Internet, ask your local library or senior center to help you locate a Web site.

Getting In-Home Help

Getting In-Home Help

Getting help with caregiving in the home involves the following options:

- **Using a home health care agency.** *In 2013, the national average hourly rate for home health aides is $21/hour; unchanged from 2012.*

- **Hiring someone privately.** *The average hourly rate for a licensed home health aide is $19 per hour and ranges from $12 to $38 per hour, depending on where in the country the services are offered, the cost of assistance is based on the category of professional need or his or her experience).*

- **Performing all caregiving duties with the assistance of family and friends.**

Use a Home Health Care Agency

Home Health Care Agencies are for-profit, nonprofit, or are run by the government. They provide personal care, skilled care, instructions for caregiver and care receiver, and supervision. They usually provide certified nurse assistants (CNAs), sometimes called home health aides; registered nurses (RNs); licensed practical nurses (LPNs); physical therapists, occupational therapists, and speech therapists. (A doctor's prescription is required in order to get coverage for skilled-care nursing in the home.) These agencies help plan services and care that match the health, social, and financial needs of the client.

Definitions for Agencies

There are a number of terms to describe an agency's services and how it is able to do what it does. Study the terms carefully before looking into the agencies in your area.

Accredited—Services have been reviewed by a nonprofit organization interested in quality home health care.

Bonded—The agency has paid a fixed dollar amount in order to be bonded. In the event of a court action the bond pays the penalties. (Being bonded does not ensure good service.)

Certified—The agency has met the lowest federal standards for care and takes part in the Medicare program.

Certified Health Personnel—Those who work for the agency meet the standards of a licensing agency for the state.

Insurance Claims Honored—The agency will look into insurance benefits and will accept assignment of benefits (meaning the insurance company pays the agency directly).

> *Tip*
>
> Ask agencies specifically about your insurance company (i.e., Blue Cross) and ask whether they have made claims to them before. Ask if there were any problems.

Licensed—The agency has met the requirements to run its business (in those states that oversee home health care agencies).

Licensed Health Personnel—The personnel (staff) of the agency have passed the state licensing exam for that profession.

Screened—References have been checked; a criminal background check may or may not have been made.

> **Tip**
>
> Beware of hiring anyone without references or a complete background check, including checking with the FBI. If you must pay for a background check, the costs maybe lower at your local Sheriff's department. Individuals who are being screened can go to the local sheriff's department to have their fingerprints scanned.

How to Pay for Using an Agency

Paying for care from an agency ranges from Medicare to private pay to long-term-care insurance to state and county programs.

Medicare

For Medicare to cover home health services, they must be "reasonable and necessary" services for the treatment of an illness or injury. If skilled nursing care on a part-time or intermittent basis is required, it must be provided by a registered nurse or a licensed practical nurse. The following services are covered under Medicare:

- Physical therapy, speech-language pathology services, and occupational therapy

- Home health aide services (like help with personal care such as bathing, using the toilet, or dressing) on a part-time or intermittent basis and medical social services (such as counseling or help finding resources in your community) if you're also getting skilled care, such as nursing care or other therapy, from the home health agency.

- Certain medical supplies, like wound dressings, that are ordered by the physician as part of your necessary care

- Durable medical equipment (like a walker, wheelchair, or other assistive device)

NOTE State rules vary on who is eligible, so check with your area Medicare office for local rules.

State and County Personal Assistance Programs

- The person receiving services may need to be certified as eligible for a nursing home.

- Many programs require that the person be at a low-income level.

- Funding may come from Medicaid waivers, and funding is sometimes limited or reduced

 Tip In most states, you maybe placed on a waiting list for these services because the need in 2013 is outpacing the available funding.

If lower income, contact your local Health and Human Services Department or the aging services division in your county where they offer a local registry of certified in-home support workers.

Private Pay

- If a person does not qualify for public funds, he or she must pay with long-term-care insurance or pay privately.

- Care management through Area Agencies on Aging may be free or offered on a sliding scale, based on a person's income.

What the Home Health Care Agency Can Do

- Carry out an in-home visit

- Look into insurance benefits and publicly funded benefits at your request

- Ask for an assignment of benefits (where payments are made by the insurer directly to the agency)

- Ask you to sign a form to release medical information

- Ask you to agree to and sign a service contract at an agreed rate

- Carry out an assessment (by the director of nurses) to determine the level of care required

- Discuss the costs of suggested services

- Come up with a plan of care that shows the person's diagnosis (what is wrong), functional limitations (what the person can and cannot do), medications, special diet, what services are provided by agency, advice for care, and list of equipment needed

- Give you a written copy of the plan of care

- Send a copy of the plan of care to the person's doctor

- Select and send the right caregivers, only to the level of care needed, to the person's home

- Adjust services to meet changing needs

Expect the Agency to:

- Be an advocate, advisor, and service planner and to share information clearly with you

- Give a full professional assessment

- Get in touch with the care receiver's doctor as part of the assessment process

- Have knowledge of long-term-care services and how to pay for them

- Fill out the paperwork for publicly funded benefits

- Show no bias or favor to service providers who may have contracts with the agency

- Provide confidential treatment that will not be talked about with others

- Provide gender-specific requests (i.e., a female may be more comfortable having a female personal care assistant).

- Provide nonjudgmental care to someone identifying with the Lesbian, Gay, Bisexual, or Transgendered (LGBT) community, assuring this will not affect care.

- Provide a written account of care when you ask for it

- Have a proven track record of being honest, reliable, and trusted if the agency handles a person's money

Tip Use caution when the agency providing the personal care assistant is also the agency handling the person's money. If personality problems arise with the care worker or there are conflicts with the agency, it is difficult to switch over financial and fiduciary responsibility to someone else, and, in some cases, it could require a court hearing if contested.

Hire Someone Privately–A Personal Assistant

Even if you decide not to use an agency, a health care professional can help you decide how to prepare the home. They can give advice about needed supplies and where to purchase them and set up a care program. However, when you hire someone privately, you must assume payroll responsibility, complete required government forms (such as Social Security), decide on fringe benefits, provide time off or vacation, decide whether overtime hours may occur and at what pay rate, track travel expenses, and provide a detailed list of tasks to be done.

Checklist Things to Do Before Selecting an Agency

✔ Interview several agencies.

✔ Get references and CHECK THEM.

✔ Make a list of services you want and ask the agency what it will cost.

✔ Ask what the steps are in the care planning and management process and how long each will take.

✔ Find out how and when you can contact the care manager.

✔ Find out if the agency has a system for sending a substitute (stand-in) aide if the regular one doesn't show up.

✔ Ask if the agency will replace the aide if that aide and the person in care do not get along.

✔ Ask about the skills and ongoing training of personnel.

✔ Ask how they keep track of the quality of services.

✔ Ask for the services needed by the person in care, even if the insurance company is trying to hold down costs.

✔ Be aware that if a social service agency is providing the care services, they may limit you to only the services that they provide.

✔ Ask them to tell you about any referral-fee agreements they may have with nursing homes or other care facilities.

✔ Know what you have to do to lodge complaints against the agency with the state ombudsman or long-term-care office.

✔ Get in touch with the local/state Division for Aging Services to check for complaints against a particular agency.

Tip

WHEN YOU START CALLING FOR RESOURCES:

- Have information ready, such as what services will be needed and personal information, such as the age of the person, date of birth, Social Security number, etc.).

- Have your questions written down and ready.

- Realize that, to be eligible for some services, there may be income, age, or geographic requirements.

- COMMUNICATE, COMMUNICATE, COMMUNICATE what you want and need!

Where to Find Help

- Yellow Pages under or Google search Nurses, Nursing Services, Aging, Independent Living, Caregiving, Social Service Organizations, Home Health Services, In-Home Support, and Senior Services

- Commercial agencies, which operate like temp employment agencies, screen applicants, and provide you with a list of candidates

- Nonprofit agencies, such as the Visiting Nurse Association, which may charge a fee on a sliding scale (based on ability to pay)

- For-profit agencies, such as the Professional Association of Geriatric Care Managers

- Public health nursing through a county social service department (if you have no insurance or money)

- Hospital discharge planner

- Hospital-based home health agencies

- School of nursing at a local community college

- College employment offices

- Hospices (call the National Hospice Organization)
- Nurses' registries
- Catholic Charities, Jewish Family Services, and other faith-based groups
- American Red Cross
- Churches, synagogues, mosques
- Nearby nursing home employee seeking part-time work
- Adult relative whom you would pay a fair hourly wage for services
- Veterans; see resources at the end of this chapter.

 In a number of states, the care receiver can hire a family member or friend to care for them.

 MONEY FOLLOWS THE PERSON
The Affordable Care Act extended the Money Follows the Person (MFP) program through 2016, giving states more options to transition Medicaid beneficiaries living in facilities back to the community. Contact your local Area on Aging for more information on home community-based services (HCBS) benefits and other caregiver support programs.

Types of Health Care Professionals

Registered Nurse (RN)—has at least 2 years of school training and is licensed by the state Board of Nursing Examiners

Licensed Practical Nurse (LPN)—has finished a one-year course of study and is licensed by the state Board of Licensed Vocational Nurses

Certified Nurses Aide (CNA)—has finished 70 hours of classes and 50 hours of clinical practice in a nursing center setting; must pass a test and register with the State Board of Nursing

Home Health Aide—is screened on the basis of work experience; training and requirements differ from state to state

Someone who is taking classes or is in a training program that leads to one of the above professions might be able to help with care.

Tax Rules You Must Follow If You Hire Privately

Most care receivers who hire an in-home support worker to perform domestic services in their home become employers. Employment taxes are due for housekeepers, companions, home health aides, and other domestic workers.

- If you pay a household employee above a certain amount (e.g. $1,800 in 2012) in a year, you are required to pay payroll taxes. Many times, this kind of tax is referred to as "nanny taxes." These taxes apply to all household employees, including housekeepers, babysitters, and elder care workers.

NOTE Some States may require you to obtain workers' compensation and disability insurance policies.

- You may use federal income tax return Form 1040-ES to pay the Social Security, Medicare, and Federal Unemployment (FUTA) taxes (employees do not have this tax withheld). Ask the Internal Revenue Service for Publication 15, Employer's Tax Guide.

- For paying Social Security tax, call the Social Security office's toll free number (800) 772-1213 or go to your local office. Look in the front of your phone book under State Government or Google on "Social Security."

How to Screen a Personal Hire

- Check licenses, training, experience, and references.

- Be sure the professional who is applying for hire has malpractice or liability insurance or is bonded.

- Run a criminal background check and a driving record check (through your local Sheriff's office and closest DMV office). Also, ask to see the person's auto insurance card.

- Find out if the person has a special skill (for example, working with care receivers who have multiple sclerosis or other neurological disorders).

- Decide whether the person is someone who can meet the emotional needs of the person in your care.

- Consider his or her personal habits, and ask is this person a personality match.

- Find out if he or she is a smoker or nonsmoker.

NOTE You can hire a private investigator to look at public records and check on education and licenses, driving history, criminal or civil charges, and previous employers. This service can be obtained anywhere in the country. If you have access to a computer, it is easy to do an instant background check search through a number of Internet providers. The cost is between $19 and $50, depending on how much information you want.

> *Tip*
>
> If you are unsure about which Internet provider to choose, go to the Consumer Affairs Web site and enter "Internet background checks" to see if there are complaints listed on the provider of interest.

Questions to Ask of the Applicant's References:

When someone is going to be hired, ask for the names of people who can tell you about this person's work and personal habits. Here are some questions you can ask:

- How long have you known this person?

- Did this person work for you?

- Is this person reliable, on time for work, patient, able to adjust as things change, able to be trusted, and polite?

- How does this person handle disagreements and emergencies?

- How well does this person follow directions, respond to requests, and take advice?

Perform All Caregiving Duties Yourself

If you decide to provide all the caregiving yourself, you can receive training at the following places:

- Social service agencies

- Hospitals

- Community schools

- American Red Cross

NOTE The National Family Caregiver Support Program offers family caregivers long-term services and supports. (Contact the National Center on Caregiving through the Family Caregiver Alliance; for information, see resources section.) If the *care receiver* is eligible:

- Adult family members or other informal caregivers age 18 and older providing care to individuals 60 years of age and older;
- Adult family members or other informal caregivers age 18 and older providing care to individuals of any age with Alzheimer's disease and related disorders;
- Grandparents and other relatives (not parents) 55 years of age and older providing care to children under the age of 10; and
- Grandparents and other relatives (not parents) 55 years of age and older providing care to adults aged 18–59 with disabilities.

Services are tailored to the type of need and hours required by a program social worker's assessment. Benefits and eligibility requirements vary from state to state and community to community.

The care receiver must also be of limited income for public benefits but check to see if your state offers a share of cost.

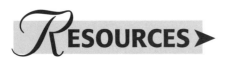

RESOURCES ➤

National Center on Caregiving, Family Caregiver Alliance
San Francisco, CA 94103
Call the National Center M-F from 9:00 A.M.–5:00 P.M.
(800) 445-8106 (voice)
(415) 434-3388 (local)

(415) 434-3508 (fax)
www.caregiver.org
info@caregiver.org
National resource center for family caregivers providing care to those with chronic disabling conditions or the elderly. The Web site provides informational fact sheets on important topics and provides services and programs in policy, education, research, and advocacy.

Caregiver Action Network (CAN)
10400 Connecticut Avenue, Suite 500
Kensington, MD 20895-3944
(800) 896-3650 (voice)
(301) 942-6430 (local)
info@caregiveraction.org
http://caregiveraction.org/
The association supports, empowers, educates, and advocates for more than 65 million Americans who care for a chronically ill, aged, or disabled person.

Veterans
Services for Family Caregivers of Post-9/11 Veterans
VA Caregiver Support Line: (855) 260-3274
http://www.caregiver.va.gov/support_benefits.asp

Home Care Agencies/Hiring Help

Council for Jewish Elderly SeniorLife
Bernard Horwich Building
3003 W. Touhy Avenue
Chicago, IL 60645
(773) 508-1000
info@cje.net
www.cje.net
Provides resources about life enrichment, supportive care resources, health care, research and education.

National Association for Home Care
228 Seventh Street, SE
Washington, DC 20003
(202) 547-7424
www.nahc.org
Provides referrals to state associations, which refer callers to local agencies. Offers publications, including the free pamphlet "How to Choose a Home Care Agency: A Consumer's Guide." Information on finding help, interviewing, reference checking, training, being a good manager, maintaining a good working and personal relationship, problems that might arise and how best to solve them, service dogs, assistive technology, and tax responsibilities.

AARP Cost of Care Calculator
www.aarp.org
Search "Cost of Care Calculator"

Publications

Avoiding Attendants from Hell: A Practical Guide to Finding, Hiring and Keeping Personal Care Attendants by June Price, Science and Humanities Press

Managing Personal Assistants: A Consumer Guide, published by Paralyzed Veterans of America. To purchase a copy, call (888) 860-7244 or download online at http://www.pva.org/site/c.ajIRK9NJLcJ2E/b.6357755/apps/s/content.asp?ct=8825357

If you don't have access to the Internet, ask your local library or senior center to help you locate a Web site.

Paying for Care

Paying for Care

*Y*ou can look to many sources for help in paying for care. Some are public, while others are private or volunteer. The most common ways to pay for home care are as follows:

- *Personal and family resources*

- *Private insurance*

- *Medicare, Medicaid, Department of Veterans Affairs, and Title programs*

- *Community based services*

- *Through trusts such as a special needs trust*

- *Personal care agreements*

 Tip Personal care agreements are financial arrangements for paying for care commonly between an adult child and his or her parent(s).

Assessment of Financial Resources

First, complete a personal financial resources assessment by doing the following steps:

- Look at current household assets, where your income comes from, and insurance entitlements.

- Prepare a budget and figure out what your future income might be from all sources.

- Confirm the qualifications, retirement benefits, and Social Security status of the person in your care.

- Figure as closely as possible the expenses of professional care and equipment. Include any medical procedures likely to be needed.

- Check on the person's personal tax status and find out what care items and expenses are deductable.

- Find out if the person's health insurance or employer's workers' compensation policy has home health care benefits.

- Figure out how much money the person will need.

 Get tax advice about making the person in your care a "dependent" and thus be able to transfer medical expenses to a taxpayer who can make use of qualifying deductions.

Caregiver Tax Considerations

1. Claim your elderly parent as a dependant.

2. The multiple support declaration exemption provides a deduction to one sibling if several are contributing to a parent's care. Every year, each sibling must sign and agree to the terms. See IRS 2120 Publication: Multiple Support Declaration.

3. Child and Dependant Care Credit: The care recipient must be claimed as a dependant. See IRS form 2441 Publication.

4. If you are not able to claim your parent as a dependant because she or he had a gross income in 2012 of more than $3,700, you may be able to deduct their medical expenses. See IRS Publication 502: Medical and Dental Expenses (including the health coverage tax credit).

> **NOTE** Keep in mind that everyone's situation is different, and tax laws and eligibility for social services benefits regularly change. For the most current advice, contact an estate planning or elder care attorney.

Public Pay Programs

Medicare

Medicare is a federal health insurance program. It provides health care benefits to all Americans 65 and older and to those younger than 65 who have been determined to be "disabled" according to the Social Security Administration. People of any age with end-stage renal disease (permanent kidney failure) requiring dialysis or kidney transplant are also covered. Those with Lou Gehrig's disease may be covered also; check with Medicare. There are constant changes in Medicare policies, requirements, and forms. Therefore, it is always best to get the most current information on benefits by calling the **Medicare Hotline** at 800-633-4227 or your hospital's social worker.

> **NOTE** You can only enroll in or make changes to your Medicare coverage during certain Initial Enrollment Periods (IEPs).

> **NOTE** When advocating for a loved one about Medicare, contact the Medicare Rights Center at (800) 333-4114.

Things That Affect Medicare Eligibility

Whether the Person Is Homebound—Medicare will pay for certain home health care services only if the person is confined to the home and requires part-time skilled (nursing) services or therapy. Medicare does not cover ongoing custodial (maintenance) care. "Confined to home" or "homebound" does not mean bedridden. The care receiver may leave home for medical treatment or short absences for nonmedical reasons, such as attending religious services. Home health care support is still possible if the person in your care attends adult day care. (Brief absences from the home do not affect eligibility.)

In order for treatments, services, and supplies to be paid, they must be ordered by a doctor. They must also be provided by a home health agency certified by Medicare and the state health department.

Whether Care Is Intermittent (periodic)—In order to be covered, skilled services are required. Medicare is not designed to meet chronic ongoing needs that are considered "custodial" rather than "skilled."

NOTE Original Medicare is the "traditional" fee-for-service program paid directly through the federal government. It means that you can see any doctor that takes Medicare, anywhere in the country. Together, Part A and Part B are called the "Original Medicare." The Medicare "Health Plan" is not "Original Medicare," so always check to see what home health benefits are covered under your plan.

Medicare Generally Pays for the Following:

- Almost all costs of skilled care, such as doctors, nurses, and specialists

- Various types of therapy—occupational, physical, speech-language

- Home health services

- Medical supplies and equipment

- Personal care by home health aides (such as bathing, dressing, fixing meals, even light housekeeping and counseling) after discharge from a hospital or nursing home

- Medical social services to help with emotional concerns related to illness

Tip

The **Affordable Care Act (ACA)** makes many improvements to Medicare, including many of the preventive services included in the "Your Medicare Benefits" booklet.

Under the ACA, you can use the Marketplace service to apply for coverage, compare options, enroll, and learn about your state's particular requirements. You can find your state's Marketplace online at https://www.healthcare.gov/what-is-the-marketplace-in-my-state/.

Open enrollment for Marketplace plans began October 1, 2013. Coverage starts as January 1, 2014.

Go to https://www.healthcare.gov/how-can-i-get-ready-to-enroll-in-the-marketplace/to sign up for e-mail or text updates to the ACA; learn about different types of health coverage; understand deductibles, out-of-pocket maximums, co-payment, and coinsurance. Before you start, gather information about your household income, set your budget, talk to your employer about health coverage. For more information, call (800) 318-2596 or TTY (855) 889-4325. The help line is open 24/7.

Medicare Part D—Prescription Drug Plan

The Medicare Part D optional plan will provide prescription drug coverage. If you have Original Medicare (Part A for hospital services and/or Part B for doctor and outpatient health-care providers), you may enroll in a stand-alone Medicare Part D prescription drug plan. This plan is run by private insurance companies, so compare types of plan coverage and out-of-pocket costs. If you cannot afford a

Prescription Drug Plan, financial help may be available. The estimated total premium is based on your income and type of plan. You may be required to pay a yearly deductible, so choose your plan carefully.

NOTE You must carry Medicare Part B (doctors visits) at a minimum to be eligible. The premium for most people is $104.90 with a deductible of $147/year.

Medicare Advantage Plans

Medicare Advantage plans are sometimes called Part C plans. These are Medicare health plans but are managed by insurance companies. Some cover prescription drug costs, dental care, and even vision care, which is not covered by Original Medicare. Also available is the Medicare Advantage Special Needs Plan (SNP) for people with specific diseases, like diabetes. The premium for an SNP will be close to what you would pay for a Medicare Advantage Plan. These plans may restrict you to only the doctors and hospitals on the managed-care provider's list. SNPs are managed by private companies that have been approved by Medicare (See **Resources**, p. 89).

NOTE If you have both Medicare and Medicaid (dual eligibility), most of your SNP needs will be covered without your paying a premium.

Help is available to pay for co-payments and premiums for those with low incomes. To be considered for dual eligibility, you must apply to the Social Security Administration for disability benefits.

Phrases like "intermittent care," "skilled care," and "homebound" are not precisely defined, and they are different from region to region. The type and availability of coverage by Medicare may be different as well.

Services NOT Covered by Medicare

Full-time nursing care at home, drugs, meals delivered to the home, homemaker chore services not related to care, and personal care services are usually not covered by Medicare.

A caregiver who has power of attorney for a person on Medicare (the beneficiary) must send written notice of this fact to the person's Medicare Part B carrier. Send a letter with the person's name, number, signature, and a statement that the caregiver can act on behalf of the beneficiary. The form must list start and end dates. If there is a dispute about a repayment from Medicare, a review can be requested by filing a claim with the Medicare carrier.

Also, keep a copy of your power of attorney document with you when conducting health, financial, or other related business on behalf of the care recipient. That way, there won't be any question as to your role.

Medicare Part B Insurance

Original Medicare stand-alone Part B insurance offers extra benefits to basic Medicare coverage. (If you have Social Security benefits, this monthly premium is automatically deducted from your benefit). Part B pays for tests, doctor's office visits, lab services, and home health care.

Medicare Supplemental Insurance (Medigap)

To pay for benefits not covered by Medicare, a "Medigap" private health insurance option is available. Medigap coverage pays for health expenses—for example, treatments, supplements, or co-pays—that Medicare does not cover. Medigap does not cover long-term care services such as a nursing facility. It does not cover dental, vision, or hearing care; eyeglasses; or private duty nursing. Most policies do not offer prescription drug coverage. Coverage and costs depend on the plan you buy. You must already be enrolled in the Original Medicare plan to be eligible to purchase Medigap insurance.

NOTE Insurance companies set premiums based on:
"Attained-Age." As you grow older, your premiums increase.

"Issue-Age." Your premium is set at your age of enrollment, but Issue-Age premiums may be increased for inflation.

"No-Age." These are the least common insurance policies based on age. Younger policy holders may pay lower premiums than older purchasers due to the higher expected health care needs of an older buyer.

For anyone who has Medicare HMO coverage, Medigap insurance may *not* be necessary because those individuals only make a small co-payment but do not pay a deductible for doctor's visits. If you are enrolled in a Medicare Advantage plan, you should not need a Medigap policy. If you have a Medigap policy and you enroll in a Medicare Advantage plan, you might lose your right to a Medigap policy. Check your state for Medigap age and disability eligibility rules.

NOTE It is illegal for anyone to sell you a Medigap policy when they know you already have one unless you put in writing that you intend to end the Medigap policy you have. It is illegal for anyone to pressure you into buying a Medigap policy or to switch insurance companies. Call Medicare at (800) 633-4227 for information on how to file a complaint.

Medicaid

Medicaid is both a federal and state insurance program. Generally, Medicaid is offered based on federal requirements, but states can change which programs they provide and what makes a person eligible. Medicaid pays for the medical care of low-income persons or those whose assets are low enough within a five-year "look-back" period. The law restricts transfers (gifts of money, stock, or other assets made to family members, etc.) made during the five years "looking back" from the date you apply for benefits. For this reason, it is wise to seek the advice of an elder law lawyer or financial planner as soon as you think you are 5–10 years away from having long-term care needs. Financial planning in this area is essential to avoid high penalties and a period of ineligibility. Eligibility depends on age (65+), personal assets, permanent disability, and citizenship status or residency. Coverage includes nursing facilities, assisted living, foster care, and certain types of home care. Keep in mind that each state runs its own Medicaid program, and so eligibility and coverage can vary. Some states have set up *Medicaid waiver programs*, which pay for home- and community-based services (HCBS waiver programs) that would otherwise only be paid if one were in a nursing home. Many states (for example, California, Florida, Texas, and Alabama) allow a family member or friend to provide paid care through the "consumer-directed care" programs, rather than someone coming from your local county in-home supportive services. To see your state benefits, go to the **Family Caregiver Alliance** Web site at www.caregiver.org to use the **Family Care Navigator**; or, call their **National Center on Caregiving** for assistance at (800) 445-8106.

 If you don't meet Medicaid's functional eligibility criteria (that is, permanent disability), then Medicaid will not pay for long-term care services, no matter how low your income is.

Common Aspects of Medicaid

- Recipients must be of limited income and disabled or blind.

- For recipients who are terminally ill, benefits go on for as long as they are ill. However, care must be provided by an agency with hospice certification and Medicaid certification.

- Payments are made directly to providers of services.

- Long-term custodial care in a nursing facility is covered for those not covered by other insurance.

- Payments to retirement communities are not covered (except in some cases by Medicaid waiver).

- Home health care services, medical supplies, and equipment are covered.

- Eligibility is based on a person's limited income and assets but varies by state.

- People with disabilities or who are blind and eligible for state public assistance are eligible for Medicaid.

- People with disabilities eligible for Supplemental Social Security (SSI) are eligible for Medicaid.

- In many states, there are laws (called spousal impoverishment laws) that protect a portion of the estate and assets for the healthy spouse. These come into play after other monies have been "spent down" for the care of the ill spouse.

NOTE In June 2013, laws were passed granting protections for same-sex couples who have married and live in states that permit same-sex marriage. Check your state for spousal impoverishment protections or other benefits concerning taxes, Social Security, or long-term care. To find out what these federal benefits are, contact your local Social Security office, city or county public assistance office, National Center on Caregiving at the Family Caregiver Alliance, or, if a senior, contact the Area Agency on Aging.

Services NOT Covered by Medicaid

As a rule, Medicaid does not cover many in-home services because they are not *medical* services. However, some community services may be called on to fill the gap for free or on a subsidized (public funding) basis. The following services usually are not covered:

- Elective or cosmetic procedures

- Medical procedures related to obesity

- Adult day care that is not for medical reasons or for those with Alzheimer's

- Alcohol and drug programs (unless they involve medical or mental health care)

- Case management (unless through a waiver program)

- Household chore services (unless through a waiver program)

- Neighborhood and local meal services, such as Meals on Wheels

- Consumer protection

- Emergency response systems (which provide contact by phone or electronic device to police and rescue services)

- Emergency assistance for food, clothing, or shelter

- Friendly visitors (volunteers who stop by to write letters or run errands)

- Services and equipment for those who have disabilities

- Homemaker services

- Legal and financial services

- Respite care (unless through a waiver program)

- Senior centers

- Support groups (which will send materials if you write to them)

- Telephone reassurance (volunteers who make calls to or receive calls from those who are elderly or living alone)

NOTE Check to see what services are offered in your state through the National Family Caregiver Support Program (Older Americans Act, Title IIIE legislation) by contacting the Eldercare Locator at (800) 677-1116.

NOTE The U.S. Congress and the Obama Administration made major changes to Medicare and Medicaid that will affect payment for long-term care. As these changes are put into effect, they are posted on the Web site of the Center for Medicare and Medicaid Services (CMS) at www.cms.gov

NOTE The Affordable Care Act (ACA) intends to provide Americans with quality, affordable health care. The ACA contains nine titles or levels of care accessed through "exchanges." Basically, under the ACA, everyone who makes above a certain income limit will help to pay for the medical care of those who fall below the poverty line.

Department of Veterans Affairs Benefits

Veterans generally qualify for health services in the home for a service-related disability. Even if a disability is not service related, other benefits may be available based on income qualifications. These services include nursing home care and at-home care for aging veterans with long-term care needs. Some states have special programs only for veterans who live in that state. Some veterans hospitals have programs

 NOTE New to veterans under the "Caregivers and Veterans Omnibus Health Services Act" of 2010 (Public Law 111-163) is the caregiver support hotline, staffed by clinical social workers with expertise in veterans caregiver resources. Under this 2011 legislation, the Veterans Administration pays for caregiving benefits to post-911 service-members.

Eligibility is generally limited to those who sustained a serious injury—including traumatic brain injury, psychological trauma, or other mental disorder—while in the line of duty on or after September 11, 2001.

Eligibility is generally based on a veteran's inability to perform one or more activities of daily living (ADLs) and need for personal care services.

For the caregiver, this new law allows a monthly payment; travel expenses; access to health insurance, mental health services, and respite time; and extensive training provided by Easter Seals. The toll free Caregiver Support Hotline is (855) 260-3274.

to deliver home health care services. Contact the nearest **Veterans Affairs** office at (800) 827-1000 or call a veterans group in your area.

Older Americans Act (OAA) and Social Services Block Grants

The OAA provides federal funds to pay for home- and community-based long-term care services (HCBS) for older adults 60+ and their caregiving families who are eligible for assistance. The purpose of these benefits is to provide care to seniors through support services in their homes, rather than in institutionalized care. Some agencies that provide support services get funding under this program. Available services may include:

- Family caregiver services and supports

- Personal care assistance for household chore services (minor household repairs, cleaning, yard work)

- Legal services that protect the rights of older persons

- Meals in a community setting

- Nutrition, such as home-delivered hot meals (Meals on Wheels) once or twice a day

- Health promotion to prevent or manage illness

- Transportation services, if available in your community and based on level of disability

Private Pay Long-Term Care Insurance

Generally, private insurance programs do not automatically cover long-term care. In many cases, home care reimbursement is severely restricted or prohibited. Policies must be examined closely. Before buying long-term care insurance (LTCI), seek the best, most knowledgeable help available on the subject (for example, consult a hospital discharge planner or the Area Agency on Aging). Seek agents who represent reliable companies and have a reputation for honesty. The lack of uniformity in long-term care policies makes it hard to compare them.

- Policies vary greatly, so don't assume one is like another you are familiar with.

- It's important to read the fine print.

- Such policies should not be considered an option for anyone over 79.

- Coverage is sometimes limited to Medicare-certified nursing homes.

- Sometimes benefits are provided for hospice care for the terminally ill.

- At age 55, after a waiting period, benefits could pay $100–150 daily for 3 years.

- A typical policy for a healthy, single 65-year-old can cost over $3,000 per year.

- Long-term care insurance should be purchased before age 60, when premiums are relatively low.

- Some companies offer direct cash payments for home care instead of reimbursement (so payment can be used for a family caregiver).

- It is important to buy what you can comfortably afford.

 For more information, visit the American Association for Long-Term Care Insurance at http://www.aaltci.org.

> **NOTE**
> LTCI has two parts:
> Long-term care includes a range of services and supports that a person needs over a period of time that are not generally medical but rather are "custodial," such as needing help with bathing, dressing, or eating.
>
> Other care supports common to long-term care are more practical, like housekeeping, preparing and cleaning up after meals, financial management, caring for pets, or shopping tasks.

To activate an LTCI policy, the policy holder must get confirmation from a qualifying medical provider that he or she has lost the ability to do two or more of the following: bathing, eating, dressing, moving without falling, going to the toilet, and moving from a bed to a chair. The insurance company may provide a representative to confirm the diagnosis. Homemaker benefits usually do not go into effect until 90 to 120 days after a hospital stay, and strict criteria must be met before in-home help is provided.

Consider Long-Term-Care Insurance If:

- Generally, personal assets (excluding a home) exceed $100,000 for a couple or $50,000 for a single person.

- The assets cannot be transferred.

- There is a family history of illness.

- You wish to protect accumulating retirement assets.

Checklist **Long-Term-Care Insurance Policies**

✓ Look for an insurer that is top rated by Moody's Investors Service, A.M. Best Company, or Standard & Poor's Corporation.

✓ Find out how long the company has been in business and check the Better Business Bureau or the state's Insurance Division for complaints.

✓ Take someone with you when you meet the agent.

✓ Never pay cash to an agent. The payment should be made by check, written to the insurance company. Be sure the agent gives you a signed and dated receipt when the policy is delivered.

✓ Find premiums that do not exceed 5–6% of the covered individual's income.

✓ Ask for an "Outline of Coverage," which the law requires the insurance company to provide even if you do not want to fill out an application for insurance. Use this outline to compare policies.

✓ Understand how and when you can contact the care manager.

✓ Look for a policy that pays for care at home, in any adult foster care home, assisted living facility, and nursing home (not just one that is Medicare certified).

✓ Avoid policies that cover only skilled care. Look for policies that allow respite care and adult day care.

✓ Find out when the insurance pays for home custodial care or hospice care.

✓ Find out if previous hospitalization, a nursing home stay, or other restrictive eligibility criteria are required.

✓ Be sure that benefits will increase with inflation.

✓ Make sure that benefits last at least 3 years if you don't buy lifetime benefits.

✓ Find out if some coverage is provided if the policy lapses and what conditions must be met before benefits can be started.

✓ Make sure the policy is guaranteed renewable regardless of age.

✓ Get several proposals before making a decision.

A younger person might consider LTCI if he can afford to protect against sudden life changes such as serious illness or a disabling accident.

A single person with no family is at higher risk of not having someone available to provide care.

 Many states license individuals to offer a cost analysis of insurance coverage. In some states, if a person has a license to sell and a license to counsel, he or she can only perform one of those services for a specific client. Check your state department of insurance for information about insurance counselors or contact the American Association for Long-Term Care Insurance.

Health Maintenance Organizations (HMOs)

Health maintenance organizations are prepaid health insurance plans that provide medical coverage for a fixed premium. Knowing whether an HMO is right for the person in your care requires careful study.

Types of HMOs

There are three types of HMOs:

- **Individual Practice Associations (IPA) Plans**—A patient chooses a doctor from a primary care physician list.

- **Preferred Provider Organization (PPO)**—Not an HMO, but another type of managed care option. A patient may visit a doctor within the provider network or outside of it. A patient may incur a share of cost, which is called a deductible or co-pay.

- **Point of Service (POS) Plans**—A combination of the HMO and PPO. Your share of the bill will be higher than if you stayed with the network provider. But a patient can visit a doctor outside of the network list without consulting her primary doctor.

Remember, HMOs receive the same fees to treat a healthy person as a person with a chronic disease. For some patients with long-term or chronic illness, HMOs may not be a good choice. A patient who has a long-established relationship with a specialist who is not a member of the HMO's network list may not be able to continue to see that specialist.

 NOTE If a Medicare health plan is not meeting the needs of the person in your care, it is not difficult to switch to another plan or to a fee-for-service program. But check for the allowable open periods of enrollment.

How To Determine If an HMO Is Right for the Person in Your Care

- Ask if the doctor or specialist the person is now seeing is in the HMO network.

- Make a checklist of the person's medical needs—special equipment, drugs, and rehabilitation options, or help with activities. Determine if these needs are covered or can be referred.

- Check if the HMO doctor has experience in dealing with a particular illness.

- Determine the specific services offered for this type of illness.

- Ask for the name of the person in the HMO offices who decides what is medically necessary.

- Ask if there is a special Plan of Care for the person's specific illness or general health care needs.

- Ask if the person will get the *best* drugs for the condition or if generic substitutes will be offered.

- Ask how many people with this type of illness are covered under the plan in your area.

- Verify that the patient may see the specialists listed in the directory, or how they can be referred to a specialist.

- Ask if the plan allows visits to specialists without a primary care doctor's referral. Ask if specialist visits will be at a higher cost.

- If a referral is required, find out how long it lasts and if a new referral is required for every visit.

- Ask what percentage of doctors on the list are board certified (have passed a special test given by the board of their specialty).

- Ask if the doctor has a financial incentive to do tests or to keep the patient from having tests or seeing a specialist.

- Ask if the plan covers visits to doctors outside the plan's referral list. (Out-of-network coverage may be limited to a certain dollar amount.)

- Ask how many doctors in the HMO specialize in geriatric care.

- If the person in your care must travel to a specific locale for extended stays, be sure the HMO allows visits to a different HMO there.

- Ask how the person will be charged if an emergency room visit is needed while traveling.

- Ask about the process for appealing a medical decision.

- Once you have decided on an HMO, get confirmation in writing regarding the items or services that are most important to the person in your care.

- Compare patient coverage for co-payments, coinsurance, deductibles, preexisting conditions, limitations on devices, medications, or access to rehabilitation.

 Use HealthCare.gov to compare care providers at: http://www.healthcare.gov/compare/index.html

How to Appeal an HMO's Decision Regarding a Medical Procedure, Prescription, or Specialist Referral

When a treatment is denied, the goal is to reverse the denial as quickly as possible. Remember that the HMO can prolong a case in court, so the goal is to resolve the case without litigation.

Attempt to resolve any conflict with the primary care physician first. They can be of great help in moving through the bureaucracy because they work in the system. Many times, they will also advocate for a treatment a patient needs.

- Call the HMO and ask for a copy of its formal appeals process. (Federal law requires HMOs to have such a process.)

- For consumer advice or support for the appeal, call the state insurance department, state health department, advocacy group for the disease, or local Area Agency on Aging.

Tip

The member representative at the other end of the line is a person, too, and being courteous always gets a better response than being viewed as irrational or disrespectful.

Community-Based Services

Many services are provided free by local or community groups. The groups are sometimes repaid by state, local, and federal governments, but often volunteers provide care services.

These services can sometimes make it possible for a person to stay at home and maintain their quality of life and independence.

Typical Services

Community-based services include:

- **Adult Day Care Centers**, which provide services ranging from health assessment to social programs that help people with dementia or those at risk for nursing home placement.

- **Nutrition Sites**, which serve meals in settings such as senior centers, housing projects, faith-based centers, or schools, and that sometimes provide transportation.

- **Meals on Wheels**, which brings nutritionally balanced meals to the home.

- **Senior Centers**, which offer a place to socialize and eat. (Often a hot meal at noontime on weekdays is the only one served.)

- **Transportation**, offered by hospitals, nursing homes, local governments, and religious, civic, or other groups. Out-of-pocket costs vary, and fees are set on a sliding scale based on ability to pay.

Do These Services Meet Your Needs?

For whatever need you have, there is most likely a program in your area to meet it. Here are some things to think about:

- Is the person the right age and income level to be eligible for the program?

- Is it necessary for the person to belong to a certain organization to be eligible?

- Is there a limit to how many times the person can use the services of the organization?

- Is the caregiver also entitled to special benefits?

If you are a grandparent taking care of young children, you may qualify for caregiver-specific benefits (age 55 or older caring for a young child).

Where to Check for Help

- Local agencies (Catholic Charities, United Way, Jewish Family and Child Services, faith-based organizations)

- Local churches, parishes, or congregations, volunteer agencies

- Local government

- City or county public assistance offices

- Health agencies (in rural areas, usually located in the county seat)

- Personal doctor

- Family services department

- Hospital discharge planner

- Insurance company where you have your policy

- Local Area Agency on Aging

- National Center on Caregiving, Family Caregiver Alliance

- Previous or current employer (may have benefits)

- Public health department

- Social Security Administration office

- State insurance commission

- Unemployment office or Web site for additional county services

- State or local ombudsman/person or advocate

The Area Agency on Aging can help find services in your community. The staff there will know whether chore services, home-delivered meals, friendly visitors, and telephone reassurance are offered free of charge or are provided on a sliding scale. Or, call the National Center on Caregiving from any U.S. state (see Resources).

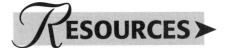 **RESOURCES**

AARP
601 E. Street, NW
Washington, D.C. 20049
(888) OUR-AARP (687-2277) (voice)
(877) 434-7598 (TTY)
(877) 342-2277 (Spanish)
www.aarp.org
Provides information on Medicare beneficiaries and caregiving.

Centers for Medicare and Medicaid Services
7500 Security Boulevard
Baltimore, MD 21244-1849
(800) MEDICARE (633-4227) Medicare Service Center (voice)
(877) 486-2048 (TTY)
www.cms.gov

www.medicare.gov
Federal agency that administers the Medicare and Medicaid programs, including hospice benefits. Online at Medicare.gov, you can also download a menu of services and file a complaint.

Family Caregiver Alliance
785 Market Street, Suite 750
San Francisco, CA 94103
(800) 445-8106
www.caregiver.org
Provides detailed information and resources across fifty states through the National Center on Caregiving (NCC). The NCC is a nonprofit service and advocacy organization that improves the lives of all older adults and community organizations.

Benefitscheckup.org
Answer some online questions to find benefit programs that can help you pay for medications, health care, food, utilities, and more. All from a reliable and trusted source.

If you don't have access to the Internet, ask your local library or senior center to help you locate a Web site.

Financial Management and Tax Planning

Financial Management and Tax Planning

There are many legal tools and tax tips that can help you and the person in your care now and in the future. Financial and life planning are necessary and should be started early. Long-term planning will help the caregiver feel more secure, no matter what the future brings. Life planning includes looking at income tax issues, protecting existing assets, saving for the future, and planning for end of life.

You should also seek advice about insurance, employment rights, and state assistance programs. If possible, discuss all options with the person in your care.

Caregivers need to understand the coverage and policies of the person in their care. This includes any medical insurance, Medicare, Medicaid, Social Security benefits, and available private disability insurance. It also means knowing about their health insurance, coinsurance, copayments, deductibles, and covered expenses.

Caregivers also need to understand the Americans with Disabilities Act (ADA), which prohibits discrimination against people with disabilities in employment, transportation, public accommodation, communications, and governmental activities.

You should get help from legal and tax experts. Laws about estate planning can be complex. This book does not cover them in detail but tells you about the tools available to you.

NOTE Financial or estate planning is simply making sure that your property—no matter how little you have—goes to the person you choose as quickly and as cost effectively as possible.

What do you do if you want to check on a financial planner's credentials before retaining him? An organization called the Financial Industry Regulatory Authority features the FINRA BrokerCheck program. This organization provides a search engine that allows you to check a broker or firm's professional background before consulting with them.

Financial Management Tools

Will—a legal document that tells who should receive which of your assets after death. If you don't have a will, the courts will decide who gets what and how much. If a person is physically unable or does not have the mental abilities (capacity) to tend to his or her own affairs, other legal papers are needed.

NOTE Make sure your designated beneficiaries are up to date and that they are those individuals you wish to receive your bequeath. Your documents are only as good as your wishes if they are prepared by the right professional and reflect your wishes at the time of a triggering incident.

Living Trust—a legal document created while you are alive rather than one created after death. This type of trust names someone (a trustee) to hold legal title to a person's property. Property left through a living trust doesn't go through probate. Not everyone needs a living trust to avoid costly and time-consuming probate court. You should consider factors such as age, single or married status, and wealth.

Power of Attorney—a written document by the principal that names someone (the agent or attorney-in-fact) to make a variety of decisions on his or her behalf. A power of attorney (POA) is either general, full, or limited to customized circumstances. Frequently, the "durable" power of attorney is used because it can continue beyond the incapacity of the principal. A person should have one power of attorney for financial management and a separate power of attorney for health care. (see **Planning End-of-Life Care**, p.107)

> **NOTE** A durable power of attorney for health care allows someone you choose to make medical decisions on your behalf if you become unable to do so. After preparing these two documents (a will and a power of attorney), you may want to include a health care directive, which is also called an advance directive, a living will, or personal directive. This way, your health and financial matters are with people you know and trust.

Representative Payee—someone named by the Social Security Administration to manage a person's Social Security benefits when that person is unable to look after his or her own money and bill paying. (Contact the Social Security Office for a full explanation of a payees roles and responsibilities.)

Conservatorship—a legal proceeding in which the court names an individual to handle another's finances when that person becomes unable to do so.

Making a will, setting up a trust, providing income, and protecting assets may involve future decisions about giving to charity, buying insurance policies, funding annuities (which make yearly payments), and creating other instruments. This kind of planning is necessary and should not be put off.

> **NOTE** Be sure to plan ahead by helping the person in your care prepare a letter of instruction. The letter should list all property and debts, location of the original will and other important documents, and names and addresses of professional advisors. It should also include funeral wishes and special instructions for giving away personal property, such as furniture and jewelry.

Income Tax Considerations

In some cases, caregivers can get income tax benefits that offset their expenses as a caregiver. If eligible, these tax "breaks" may include claiming the person in care as a dependent and receiving a "dependent care credit." For a person who is elderly or disabled, certain tax credits also apply, and some expenses are deductible.

When a Person Qualifies As a Dependent for Income Tax Purposes

A husband and wife or married same-sex partner must legally pay for each other's necessary health care, but their adult children or other relatives do not have to. However, sometimes adult children and relatives provide money or resources that will allow them to claim the person in their care as a dependent for income tax purposes, making that person's costs a deduction.

According to the IRS, there are five tests for a person to qualify as a dependent for tax purposes:

1. **IRS gross income test:** The person does not earn more than a specified amount of gross income, adjusted each year to match the personal exemption. In recent years, the gross income earned by your elderly parent had to be less than $3,800. This amount generally does not include income from disability income, but does include withdrawals from retirement plans, pension benefits, rental or property income, or other dividends.

2. **Age test:** The caregiver exemption does not apply to a child under 19 (or 24 if attending school full time).

3. **The IRS taxpayer support test:** You must show that you provide over one-half of the person's support. This is difficult to determine but includes, for example, the cost of food, transportation, clothing, housing, and medical care.

4. **The IRS relationship test:** The person receiving care has one of the following relationships with the taxpayer:

- Child

- Brother or sister

- Parent or grandparent

- Aunt, uncle, niece, or nephew

- Son-in-law, daughter-in-law, father-in-law, mother-in-law, brother-in-law, sister-in-law

- A descendant of a child (grandchild, great-grandchild)

- Stepchild, stepbrother, stepsister, or stepparent

In prior years if your elderly parent's income was over $3,800, you were still able to get a tax savings on your tax return by deducting their medical expenses (consult IRS Form 502, for eligible medical care) along with your own expenses and those of dependents.

Additional Considerations/Tests

The following are additional issues that the IRS considers to determine eligibility:

- The person lives in the taxpayer's home during the entire tax year and is a member of the taxpayer's household.

- The person did not file a joint return with a spouse.

- The person is a citizen, national, or resident of the United States, or a resident of Canada or Mexico at some time during the calendar year, or is an alien child adopted by and living with a U.S. citizen.

Tax Credit for Those Who Are Elderly or Disabled

A tax credit may be available to persons who are 65 or over. It may be available to those who are permanently or totally disabled. Special rules apply for figuring out the amount of the credit. See IRS Schedule R (Form 1040) or Schedule 3 (Form 1040A).

NOTE Some life insurance policies provide tax-free benefits (accelerated death benefits), where the benefits are paid before death. Check with the life insurance company for details.

What Can Be Deducted for Income Tax Purposes

If a person can be claimed as a dependent, and the caregiver itemizes, the caregiver may include medical expenses for the dependent on the caregiver's schedule of itemized deductions. If all medical expenses of the caregiver exceed 7.5% of the adjusted gross income, a deduction will be allowed.

Medical expenses include such things as acupuncture, adaptive devices, ambulance fees, artificial limbs, bandages, braille books and magazines, special adaptive equipment for vehicles, chiropractic care, eyeglasses, hearing aids, in-home health care services, insulin, prescription drugs, diagnostic devices, dental care, and dentures.

Other deductible medical expenses include:

- Improvements and additions to the home that are made for medical care purposes. (These are deductible only to the extent that they exceed the value added to the house. The entire cost of an improvement that does not increase the value of the property is deductible.)

- Expenses related to a service dog for a qualifying disability, such as blindness or deafness.

- Lodging while away from home for (and essential to) medical care, per person per night. Meals are not deductible.

- Premiums paid for Medicare Part B under the Social Security Act relating to supplementary medical insurance for the aged.

- Co-pays, and deductibles fort health insurance, dental and eye insurance, long-term care insurance.

- Lifetime care fees (percentage of fees paid under a lifetime care contract with a continuing care retirement community).

- Nursing facility and assisted living costs.

- Nursing services.

- Psychiatric care.

- Transportation costs to receive medical care, mileage, parking fees, and tolls.

See your tax preparer for rules about your exact situation. The rules are very complex and depend on each individual's situation. Now you know what to look for and what questions to ask.

STORING DOCUMENTS

Store—Death certificates, military records, tax returns for the past six years, pension documents

Keep in the safe-deposit box—Original will, deeds, passport, stock and bond certificates, birth and marriage certificates, insurance policies

Keep at home—A copy of the will that is in the safe-deposit box or other private and secure location

Throw out—Expired insurance policies, checks that are more than one year old and are not tax-related

Don't forget that you must tell someone you trust where these documents are and who has them.

Funeral Expenses

Funeral expenses are not usually deducted for income tax purposes but are deducted if an estate tax return is filed. If your loved one is a veteran, you may be entitled to burial costs.

Year-End Tax Tips for Family Caregivers

As early as possible, consider the following money-saving strategies and, if appropriate, discuss them with the person in your care.

- Pay or charge medical expenses in the year when the deduction will result in a benefit. Consider "bunching" medical deductions in one year (for example, buy January's prescription drugs in December).

- See if you qualify as head of household on the tax form.

- Consider transferring to a beneficiary title to the property that belongs to the person in your care. This makes sense when the beneficiary could claim expenses, such as real estate taxes, that the person in care could not claim because of a low income level. But be aware that, under Medicaid, this will disqualify you unless it's done five years *before* you apply for Medicaid, in most states.

- Determine who should pay medical bills by figuring out who will receive a tax deduction from the payment.

- Before selling assets to care for a parent, consider the tax that will have to be paid on the sale. Decide which assets have a *high* or *low basis* (original purchase price) because capital gains should be kept low. Consider gifting to the person receiving care first, then having that person sell the gift at a lower tax rate.

- Consider giving property to a charity—and doing so in a way that provides a higher income each year than he or she would receive from interest on an investment.

> ## *Tip*   TRACKING TAX-RELATED EXPENSES
>
> - Use a file box for storage.
> - Set up a separate accordion-style folder with tabs for each doctor, lab, or hospital and medicines.
> - Keep all bills in the proper folder filed by month.
> - Note the check number, date, and amount paid on each bill. (To keep better records, pay medical bills by check and not by credit card.)
> - Keep a daily diary of cash expenses, mileage, and other travel costs for medical visits. Hand-held-devices, such as a Palm Pilot, are useful for keeping this information.

Social Security Benefits

The Social Security Administration runs two federal disability retirement programs: Social Security Disability Insurance (SSDI), which is based on earned income, and Supplemental Security Income (SSI), which is for those with low incomes. SSDI is an insurance program that is funded by taxes from employees and employers. SSI is an assistance program for people with low incomes. The medical requirements and disability standards are the same, but scrutiny may be higher on attaining SSI benefits because it is coming from taxpayers investments rather than from money earned through work. Check with your local Independent Living Center's benefits counselor if you have questions about eligibility or call the Social Security Administration.

Social Security considers a person disabled when he or she is unable to perform any paid job, and the disability is expected to last for 12 months.

At full retirement age (FRA), you may begin receiving full benefits, and no earnings limits apply. You can go on line or call the **Social Security Administration** (800-772-1213) to get a report of your benefits record.

Generally, with a disability, you can earn up to $900 per month and keep your Social Security benefits, as long as you report your earnings. Social Security has an interest in getting people off reliance on the program when possible, and it offers an education or work program.

 Social Security Retirement Benefits are tax free for the majority of individuals, and partially free for the rest.

Understanding Social Security

- Retirement checks are loosely tied to how much a person paid into the system or based on eligible disability.

- If the person receiving Social Security dies, Social Security Survivor Benefits may be available to that person's spouse, widows, widowers, children, and dependent parents. See the Social Security Survivor benefits book or call the Social Security office.

- The monthly Social Security benefit typically paid to a retired worker is $1,230. The amount changes based on the total amount of benefits paid and the total number receiving benefits.

- Social Security, personal savings, investments, and employer pensions together can provide financial support in old age.

NOTE Name the personal representative as co-renter of the safe-deposit box if the person in your care does not have a spouse or close relative. This will make it easier to get into the safe-deposit box after the person's death.

Medicaid Guidelines

The cost of nursing home care is high and can easily wipe out a couple's savings, even if only one person is in a nursing home.

> **NOTE** The Affordable Care Act (ACA) expands Medicaid eligibility to 133% of the federal poverty rate. This means that the income level cutoff for a family of four is $29,700, rather than $22,350. This part of the ACA goes into effect on January 1, 2014, but is subject to policy change.

Currently, Medicaid rules allow a person:

- To keep a home if he or she plans to return there or if it is lived in by a spouse or a disabled or minor child

- To have a maximum individual income (which varies state to state), including pension payments and Social Security benefits

- To have a prepaid funeral fund of $1,500

- To have a bank account of no more than $2,000

General Points Regarding Asset Transfers

- Transfers must happen at least five years before applying to a Medicaid-financed nursing facility. (Transfers within five years may delay eligibility for Medicaid and cause penalties.)

- A home can be transferred outside the five-year period if it is transferred to a spouse, a minor, or a disabled child meeting certain conditions.

- Transfers of assets to a child may be risky if the child will not be able or willing to help the parent if extra money is later needed. A trust may be a better option because the money is still available for the parents' needs.

- If a person sets up a special-needs trust for himself, the assets must still be spent down to qualify for Medicaid payment for nursing home care.

- Among the penalties for people who transfer assets for less than fair market value to qualify for Medicaid is a $10,000 fine and up to a year in prison.

- The healthy spouse of a person who applies for Medicaid may retain some income and resources. Each case is assessed after the applicant becomes eligible for Medicaid.

- The most individual income a person can have and still get Medicaid varies from state to state. The rules can be tricky, so seek the advice of an attorney or online on the Medicaid Web site.

Employment Planning

Employment planning and retirement tips are very important. There are many issues to look into once the care receiver can no longer work. You will need to look at sick leave, short-term disability insurance, and the Family Medical Leave Act. When the person in your care decides to stop working, you will need to look into options for medical coverage. Applying for long-term disability and Social Security benefits can take a lot of time. You will need to find out what you can do while waiting for these new benefits to arrive.

You will also need to think about tapping into other sources of income once you decide to leave work. In addition to applying for Social Security or veterans benefits, you should know the cash value of your life insurance and long-term care insurance policies, and the value of personal property, real estate, and mortgage insurance.

Abuse by Financial Advisors

Aggressive marketing to the elderly is becoming increasingly common. Although seminars for estate planning can provide useful information, they are often selling something and therefore do not offer an unbiased assessment of what a person may need. Help the person in your care avoid financial planners who may also be stock brokers or insurance agents. Before selecting a financial planner, one should always:

- Check with the local Area Agency on Aging and other agencies that work with the elderly for a list of referrals.

- Interview the financial planner and check his or her credentials (law, accounting degrees, continuing education in financial planning for the retired).

- Find out what the financial advisor will gain from your business in fee and commission income.

- Check with your local senior center for recommendations.

- Take this information into account before deciding to buy.

- Ask for the fees in writing; ask for help if you don't understand them.

- Ask if local law requires that any comparisons of plans be provided.

- Ask if the advisor is registered with the Securities and Exchange Commission. (📖 See **Consumer Fraud**, p. 259)

Neither the authors nor the publisher are engaged in providing legal or tax services. This *Guide* is for general information only. In order to learn more about these matters, consult a CPA, attorney, or other professional advisor.

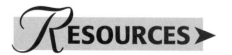

RESOURCES ➤

AARP Tax-Aide
(888) 227-7669
http://www.aarp.org/findtaxhelp (for a listing of site locations)
Call or go to the Web site between February 1 and April 15 to

find a site near you. Provides free help on federal, state, and local tax returns to middle- and low-income persons aged 60 and older. The Tax-Aide also provides online counselors at this Web site. This program also accepts volunteers.

Certified Financial Planners Board of Standards

1425 K Street, NW, #500
Washington, DC 20005
(800) 487-1497 (toll-free)
(202) 379-2200
mail@cfpboard.org
http://www.cfp.net/
This organization will provide information on whether a planner is certified, how long he or she has been certified, and if any disciplinary action has been taken.

Financial Planning Association

7535 E. Hampden Avenue, Suite 600
Denver, CO 80231
(800) 322-4237
(303) 759-0749 (fax)
Member.Services@FPAnet.org
www.fpanet.org
This Web site provides a list and gives the backgrounds of certified financial planners in your region and offers several helpful, free brochures and guides, including "How a Financial Planner Can Help You… and How to Choose the Right One," which provides tools for choosing a financial planner.

IRS Web Site

For answers to tax questions:
(800) 829-1040 (voice)
(800) 829-4059 (TDD)
www.irs.gov
The Web site provides tax forms. Form 559 is for survivors, and Form 524 is for those who are elderly or disabled.

National Association of Personal Financial Advisors
3250 North Arlington Heights Road, Suite 109
Arlington Heights, IL 60004
(888) FEE-ONLY (333-6659)
(847) 483-5400
info@napfa.org
www.napfa.org

Older Women's League
1625 K Street, NW, Suite 1275
Washington, DC 20006
(202) 567-2606
info@owl-national.org
www.owl-national.org

Paralyzed Veterans of America
www.pva.org
"Keys to Managed Care: A Guide for People with Physical Disabilities" is available at the Web site.

Social Security Administration
(800) 772-1213 (voice)
(800) 325-0778 (TTY)
www.socialsecurity.gov

Society of Financial Service Professionals
www.financialpro.org

MyMedicare.gov
An interactive Medicare portal containing personalized information regarding claims, plans and coverage, benefits, and entitlements.

Home Equity Advisor – National Council on Aging
http://www.homeequityadvisor.org/

If you don't have home access to the Internet, ask your local library or senior center to help you locate any Web site.

Planning for End-of-Life Care

Planning for End-of-Life Care

*I*n addition to deciding how to pay for long-term care and estate planning (topics covered in the past two chapters), it is important to decide how future health care decisions will be made before things reach the crisis stage. These decisions should be recorded in legal documents for two reasons:

- *To make sure that a person's wishes are honored*

- *To make sure the family has enough information about those wishes in order to make life-and-death decisions*

The ability to plan for health care decisions depends on one's ability to:

- *Understand the available treatment choices*

- *Understand the results of those options*

- *Make and communicate a thoughtful choice*

- *Express values and goals*

- *Think in terms of legal options or what's needed in protections regarding care*

Once these matters are understood, a range of legal documents can be drawn up to help ensure that the person's wishes will be carried out.

The following information is not intended as legal advice. Here, we present a general summary of the rights of capable adults to make, or arrange for others to make, their health care decisions. Our summary does not contain all the technical details of laws in each state. Check what your state requires by law.

Directives for Health Care

There are two significant types of legal documents for indicating a person's wishes if he or she is not able to make his or her own decisions. One type outlines the kind of medical attention the person wants, and the other names the person who will make sure these wishes are carried out. (The names of the documents may be different in your state.)

Living Will

A living will spells out a person's wishes about medical care in case he or she is physically unable to state those wishes. When drawing up a living will, it is important to consider a person's attitudes and desires regarding health care. (📖 See *Special Challenges*, p. 270, for having one's wishes honored while traveling.)

Health Care Proxy (Health Care Power of Attorney or Advance Directive)

This document allows a person to name someone as a personal representative (the health care proxy or representative) and gives that person the authority, or right, to carry out the person's wishes, as outlined in the living will.

Do Not Resuscitate Order (DNR)

This document instructs medical personnel not to use CPR (cardiopulmonary resuscitation) if the person's heart stops beating.

Values History Form

This document explains a person's views on life and death and what he or she thinks is important. This can help the proxy or representative understand the person's wishes.

It is a very helpful document because there is no way of knowing every medical situation that can possibly happen. The values history form will express your attitude toward your feelings about heath care providers, independence or control, personal relationships, and religion and beliefs.

Why It Makes Sense to Prepare Directives

- They can be flexible and tailored to an individual's wishes.

- They apply to all health care situations.

- They may be given to anyone—a friend, relative, or spiritual advisor—to hold until needed.

- They are honored in the state where they were written and in most other states (check the state in question).

- They are not limited to issues of prolonging life but can also, for example, cover dental work and surgery.

- They can be created by filling out a standard form.

- They can be revoked (cancelled) at any time as long as the person is mentally able.

Advance Health Care Directive forms differ from state to state and are available from most hospitals and nursing homes.

> *Tip*
>
> It is important to have access to these legal and health care documents for the person you are caring for. It is also important that you, the caregiver, have these documents drawn up for yourself.

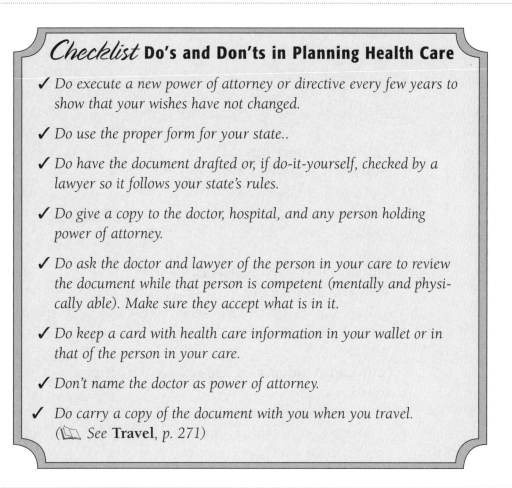

Checklist **Do's and Don'ts in Planning Health Care**

✓ *Do execute a new power of attorney or directive every few years to show that your wishes have not changed.*

✓ *Do use the proper form for your state..*

✓ *Do have the document drafted or, if do-it-yourself, checked by a lawyer so it follows your state's rules.*

✓ *Do give a copy to the doctor, hospital, and any person holding power of attorney.*

✓ *Do ask the doctor and lawyer of the person in your care to review the document while that person is competent (mentally and physically able). Make sure they accept what is in it.*

✓ *Do keep a card with health care information in your wallet or in that of the person in your care.*

✓ *Don't name the doctor as power of attorney.*

✓ *Do carry a copy of the document with you when you travel. (📖 See* **Travel***, p. 271)*

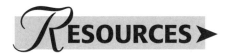

ℛESOURCES ➤

American Association of Retired Persons – Tool Kits
Health Decisions Resources
ABA Commission on Law and Aging
www.AmericanBar.org
Search "Consumer's Tool Kit for Healthcare Advance Planning".

AARP

(800) 424-3410

www.aarp.org

The AARP can direct you to a telephone hotline, available in some states, for brief legal advice to those 60 and older.

Caring Connections

(800) 658-8898 (multilingual)

www.caringinfo.org

Distributes state-specific forms and explanatory guides for creating a living will.

The Equal Justice Network

www.equaljustice.org

A Web site sponsored by programs in the field offering legal advice over the telephone.

National Academy of Elder Law Attorneys

www.naela.org

Provides a list of member lawyers in your area, plus information on veterans, disabilities, nursing homes, Medicare, and Social Security from a legal perspective.

Call your local **Social Security Administration, State Health Department, State Hospice Organization,** or call *the* **Medicare Hotline** at (800) 633-4227 to learn about hospice benefits. You might also contact your local Office of Senior Affairs, your State or Area Agency on Aging, agencies providing Legal Services for the Elderly, or your personal attorney.

If you don't have access to the Internet, ask your local library or senior center to help you locate any Web site.

Preparing the Home

Preparing the Home

Adapting the home for a person who is partially or fully disabled can be a difficult process or a simple process. In general, the more adaptations (changes) that can be made early on—with a view toward future needs—the easier life will be for everyone concerned. Few caregivers can afford to remodel a home totally. Yet, it is important for readers to be aware of the "ideal" as they plan the changes that make sense for their situations.

Here, we present suggestions—from architects who specialize in elder care housing, occupational therapists, and others—for setting up the best home care conditions.

Safety, Safety, Safety

NOTE The death rates from falls among older men and women have risen sharply over the past decade. In 2010, 2.3 million nonfatal fall injuries among older adults were treated in emergency departments, and more than 662,000 of these patients were hospitalized. Those who survive falls frequently sustain hip fractures and head injuries that result in permanent disability and reduced quality of life. (Source: Centers for Disease Control and Prevention, 2013).

The main concern in any home is safety. Accidents can happen, but with a little planning falls can be prevented. Take a close look at the home where you will provide care. You may want to ask a relative or friend to look at it with you to make sure you haven't overlooked any safety hazards.

You can also rely on a social workers assessment if you have a care plan.

 NOTE A care receiver who spends time alone should always have a cell phone in her pocket to call someone if she gets into an unsafe situation. There are many fall alert systems on the market, find the best one for you.

As you plan for safety in the home, think about what you will need now and what you will need in the future. For example, furniture that works well for a 65-year-old may need to be changed or replaced later as the person loses strength. Your first concern is to make the home as safe as possible.

As you make changes to the home, don't forget your own comfort and ease. Making life easier for yourself means you will have more time to provide care or to rest. In the long run, this will improve the overall setting for care. (See also *The Comfort of Home® for Alzheimer's Disease.*)

The Home Setting

The ideal home for the care of elderly or disabled persons is on one level (ground floor). Having more than one floor is all right, as long as there is an elevator or other approved lift device. The ideal care home is laid out so that the caregiver and the person in care can hear each other from other rooms.

Safety

For the safest home, follow as many of these steps as possible:

• Remove any furniture that is not needed, clutter is dangerous.

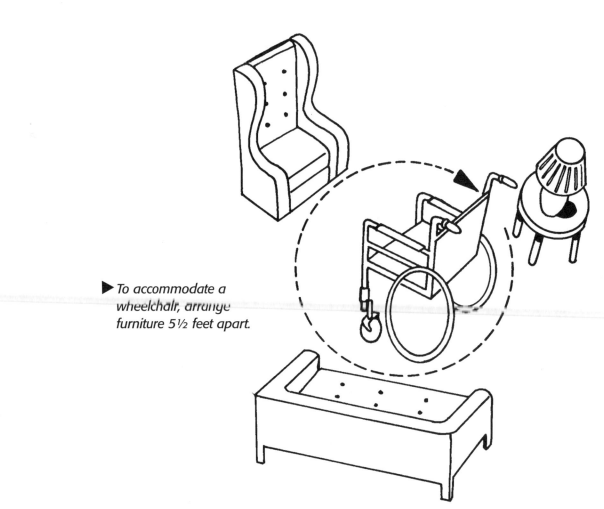

▶ *To accommodate a wheelchair, arrange furniture 5½ feet apart.*

- Place the remaining furniture so that there is enough space for a walker or wheelchair. This will avoid the need for an elderly or disabled person to move around coffee tables and other barriers. Move any low tables that are in the way.

- Once the person in your care has gotten used to where the furniture is, do not change it.

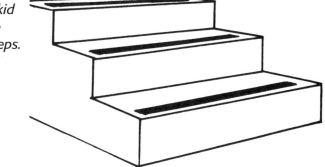

▶ *Place nonskid tape on the edges of steps.*

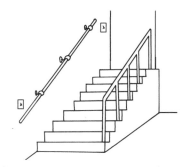

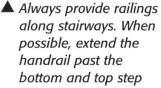

▲ *Always provide railings along stairways. When possible, extend the handrail past the bottom and top step*

- Make sure furniture will not move or break if it is leaned on.

- Make sure the armrests of a favorite chair are long enough to help the person get up and down.

- Add cushioning to sharp corners on furniture, cabinets, and vanities.

- Avoid using glass tables.

- Make chair seats 20 inches high. (Wood blocks or a wooden platform can be placed under large, heavy furniture to raise it to this level.) The chair must be easy to get out of.

- Have a carpenter install railings in places where a person might need extra support. (Using a carpenter can ensure that railings can bear a person's full weight and will not give way.)

- Place plastic decorative stickers or colored tape on glass doors and picture windows.

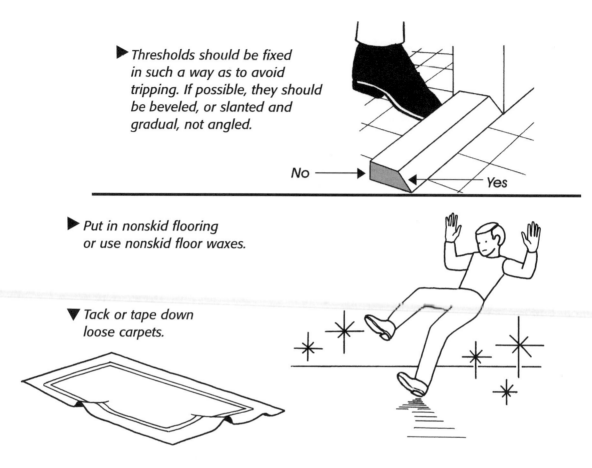

▶ *Thresholds should be fixed in such a way as to avoid tripping. If possible, they should be beveled, or slanted and gradual, not angled.*

No ⟶

Yes

▶ *Put in nonskid flooring or use nonskid floor waxes.*

▼ *Tack or tape down loose carpets.*

- Have a lamp and automatic night-lights in the rooms used by the person in your care.

- Clear fire-escape routes.

- Provide smoke alarms on every floor and outside every bedroom (see your local laws on requirements).

- Place a fire extinguisher in the kitchen, but make sure it is the correct one for household fires.

- Think about using monitors and intercoms.

- Place nonskid tape on the edges of stairs (and consider painting the edge of the first and last step a different color from the floor).

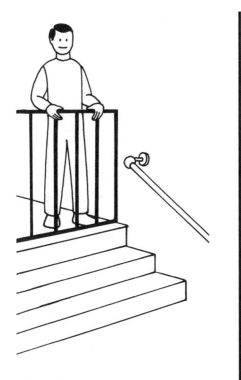

▲ *A safety gate at the top of stairs can prevent falls.*

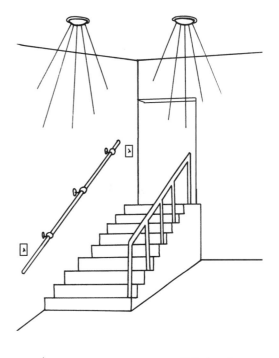

▲ *Be sure steps are well lighted with light switches at both the top and bottom of the stairs.*

- Remove area throw rugs; even using backing tape is not a guarantee of safety.

- Install light switches inside doorways so you don't walk through a dark room to turn on a lamp.

- It is easier to walk on thin-pile carpet than on thick-pile. Avoid busy patterns.

- Be sure stairs have even surfaces with no metal strips or rubber mats to cause tripping.

- Remove all hazards that might lead to tripping.

- Keep electrical and telephone cords secured and out of the way.

NOTE For a safer home setting for the person with a respiratory condition such as asthma, emphysema, or chronic bronchitis, avoid—

- Rugs
- Pleated lampshades
- Belt-type humidifiers
- Dirty heat ducts and air filters
- Overstuffed furniture

- Books and bookshelves
- Tobacco smoke
- Pets and stuffed toys
- Wool blankets and clothing

- Adjust or remove rapidly closing doors.

- Place protective screens on fireplaces

- Cover exposed hot-water pipes.

- Provide enough no-glare lighting—indirect is best.

- Place light switches next to room entrances so the lights can be turned on before entering a room. Consider "clap-on" lamps beside the bed.

- Use 100 to 200–watt light bulbs for close-up activities (but make sure lamps can handle the extra wattage).

NOTE An 85-year-old needs about three times the amount of light a 15-year-old needs to see the same thing. Contrasting colors play a big part in seeing well. As much as possible, the color of furniture, toilet seats, counters, etc., should be different from the floor color.

- Plan for extra outdoor lighting for good nighttime visibility, especially on stairs and walkways.

- If possible, install a carbon monoxide (CO) detector that sounds an alarm when dangerous levels of CO are reached. Call the **American Lung Association** (800) LUNG USA, for details.

- Have an emergency escape plan in case of fire.

- Create a disaster plan. Give each family member a copy. Have an earthquake and natural disaster safety kit to cover you for at least three days. It should include a battery/hand crank radio.

> **NOTE** If the person in your care is on life support equipment, install a backup electrical power system and have a plan of action in case the power goes out.

Comfort and Convenience

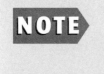

- For persons who are frail or wheelchair-bound, put in automatic door openers.

- For a person with a wheelchair or a walker, allow at least 18–24" clearance from the door on landings.

▲ *Think about getting a power-assisted recliner that allows the power-assist feature to be turned off.*

▶ *Install entry ramps. Rails can be added for more safety.*

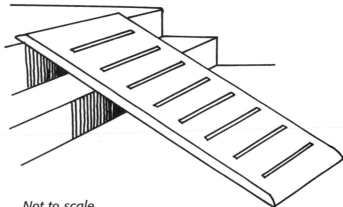

Not to scale.

• Plan to leave enough space (a minimum of 32" clear) for moving a hospital bed and wheelchair through doorways.

> **NOTE** If you are redoing or building a new two-story house, have the contractor frame in the shell of the elevator and then add the elevator unit later when needed. Use the space as a closet for now.

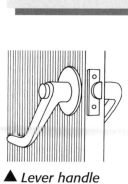

▲ *Lever handle*

• To widen doorways, remove the molding and replace regular door hinges with offset hinges. Whenever possible, remove doors.

• Put lever-type handles on all doors.

• If a person who is disabled must be moved from one story to another, install a stair elevator or lift seat.

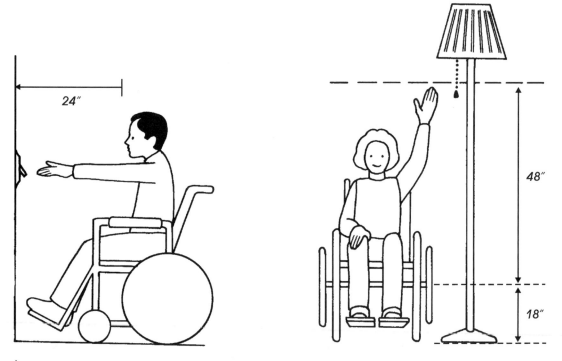

▲ *A person can reach forward about 24" from a seated position. Between 18" and 48" from the floor is the ideal position for light switches, telephones, and mail boxes.*

The Bathroom

Many accidents happen in bathrooms, so check the safety of the bathroom that you will use for home care.

Safety

▶ *Install grab bars beside the toilet, along the edge of the sink, and in the tub and shower according to the needs of each person.*

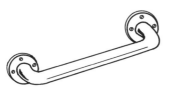

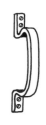

▶ *Five-inch door pulls or utility handles can be put on door frames and window sills.*

- Cover all sharp edges with rubber cushioning.

- Put lights in the medicine cabinets so mistakes are not made when taking medications.

- Remove locks on bathroom doors.

- Use nonskid safety strips or a nonslip bath mat in the tub or shower.

- Think about putting a grab bar on the edge of the vanity. (Do not use a towel bar.)

- Install grab bars in showers.

- Remove glass shower doors or replace them with unbreakable plastic or tempered safety glass.

- Place a bath and shower seat in the tub or shower.

- Use only electrical appliances with a ground fault interrupted (GFI) feature.

- Install GFI electrical outlets.

- Set the hot water thermostat below 120° F.

- Use faucets that mix hot and cold water, or paint hot water knobs/faucets red.

- Insulate (cover) hot water pipes to prevent burns.

- Put in toilet guard-rails or provide a portable toilet seat with built-in rails. (📖 See *Equipment and Supplies*, p. 139)

Comfort and Convenience

- If possible, the bathroom should be in a straight path from the bedroom of the person in your care.

- Put in a ceiling heat lamp.

- Place a telephone handset near the toilet, or take a cell phone with you.

- Provide soap-on-a-rope or put a bar of soap in the toe of a nylon stocking and tie it to the grab bar.

- Place toilet paper within easy reach.

- Try to provide enough space for two people at the bathroom sink.

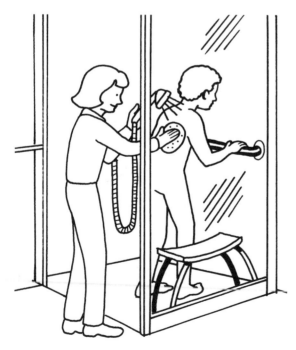

- If possible, have the sink 32–34" from the floor.

- Use levers instead of handles on faucets.

- Provide an elevated (raised) toilet seat.

◀ *If possible, have a shower stall that is large enough for two people. Use a hand-held shower head with a very long hose and adjustable jet stream. Put a tub seat or bench in the shower stall.*

The Kitchen

Many of the following suggestions are made to fit the needs of people who are handicapped or elderly who are able to help in the kitchen.

Safety

- Use an electric teakettle.

- Set the water-heater temperature at 120°F.

- Use a single-lever faucet that can balance water temperature.

- Provide an area away from the knife drawer and the stove where the person in your care can help prepare food.

- Use a microwave oven whenever possible (but not if a person with a pacemaker is present).

- Ask the gas company to modify your stove to provide a gas odor that is strong enough to alert you if the pilot light goes out.

- If possible, have the range controls on the front of the stove.

- Provide a step stool, never a chair, to reach high shelves.

▲ *Cover the floor with a nonslip surface or use a nonskid mat near the sink, where it may be wet.*

Comfort and Convenience

- Use adjustable-height chairs with locking casters.

- Install a Lazy Susan® (swivel plate) in corner cabinets.

- Set up cabinets to reduce bending and reaching.

- Put in a storage wall rather than upper cabinets.

- For easy access, replace drawer knobs with handles.

► Use "reachers"—devices for reaching objects in high or low places without stretching, bending, or standing on a stool.

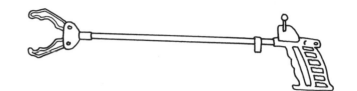

► A cutting board placed over a drawer provides an easy-to-reach surface for a person in a wheelchair.

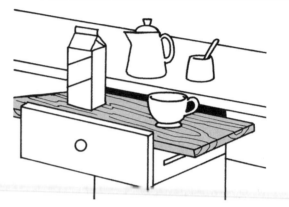

- Place a wire rack on the counter to reduce back strain from reaching dishes.

- Adapt one counter for wheelchair access as pictured above.

- Remove doors under the sink to allow for wheelchair access; also cover exposed pipes.

- Create different counter heights by putting in folding or pull-out surfaces.

- If bending is difficult, consider a wall oven.

- Use suspension systems for heavy drawers.

- Put pullout shelves in cabinets.

- If possible, use a fridge that has the freezer on the bottom.

- Prop the front of the fridge so that the door closes by itself. (If necessary, reverse the way the door swings.)

 NOTE To reduce the chance of falls and to avoid reaching and bending, place frequently used items at a level between the shoulders and knees.

The Bedroom

Ideally, provide three bedrooms—one for the person in care, one for yourself, and one for the home health aide. Also:

- Put in a monitor to listen to activity in the room of the person in your care. (Most are inexpensive and are portable.)

- Make the bedroom bright and cheerful.

- Make sure enough heat (65°F at night) and fresh air are available through a safe means, such as a window that is secured.

- Provide an appropriate mattress; ask your doctor or physical therapist.

- Provide TV and radio.

- Think about having a fish tank for fun and relaxation.

- Use throwaway pads to protect furniture.

- Install blinds or shades that darken the room.

- Place closet rods 48" from the floor.

- Provide a chair for dressing.

- Keep a flashlight at the bedside table.

- Provide a bedside commode with a 4" foam pad on the seat for comfort.

- Hang a bulletin board with pictures of family and friends where it can be easily seen.

- Provide a sturdy chair or table next to the bed for help getting in and out of bed.

- Make the bed 22" high and place it securely against a wall. Or use lockable wheels. This will allow the person to get up and down safely.

- Use blocks to raise a bed's height, but be sure to make them steady so they don't move.

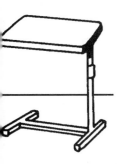

...ovide an adjustable ...er-the-bed table ...e the ones used ...serve meals in ...ospital rooms.

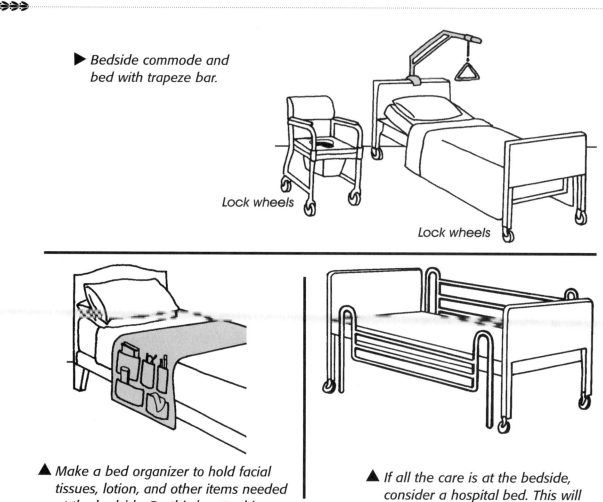

▶ *Bedside commode and bed with trapeze bar.*

Lock wheels

Lock wheels

▲ *Make a bed organizer to hold facial tissues, lotion, and other items needed at the bedside. Do this by attaching pockets to a large piece of fabric spread across the bed.*

▲ *If all the care is at the bedside, consider a hospital bed. This will be helpful for both you and the person in your care.*

The Telephone

Call your local phone company's special-needs department or visit a store that sells phones and related products. Inquire about

- Increasing the size of the numbers on your phone dial so they can be seen and used more easily

- A phone cradle

- Step-by-step, large-size instructions for using the phone

- Handsets with amplifiers that will make it easier to hear

- Signal devices, such as lights that flash when a call is coming in

▶ *Telephone with enlarged numbers*

- TTY (text telephone yoke), a telephone device for the hard of hearing

- A portable or cell phone (to keep out of reach of a person who has cognitive impairments such as dementias.)

- Speed-dial buttons with names or pictures of friends and family instead of numbers

- A one-line phone that automatically connects to a preset number when the button is pressed

- A list of emergency numbers and a list of medicines beside the telephone (📖 See **Setting Up a Plan of Care**, p. 169, for a sample.)

- Clear instructions on how to direct emergency personnel to the street address, apartment, or house where you are located

- A personal emergency response alert system to signal a friend or emergency service

NOTE Some communities provide a free **telephone reassurance service**. TRS will make a brief, daily telephone call to persons who are elderly or disabled to reassure them and to share crime prevention information. Call your local police department or the Area Agency on Aging.

Outdoor Areas

Safe outdoor areas are important, especially for those who are frail or elderly and are mobile. Safety features should include the following:

- Ramps for access on ground that is not level or even

- A deck with a sturdy railing

- Alarmed or locked outside doors

- A key hidden outside

- Enough light to see walkway hazards at night

- Nonslip step surfaces in good repair

- Stair handrails fastened to their fittings

- Step edges marked with reflective paint

- A hedge or fence around the yard and dangerous areas like pools or streams

Avoid gravel or rock yards or paths. In addition, unplug or remove power tools and other hazards.

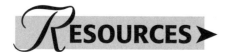

RESOURCES ➤

National Safety Council
nsc.org or email for information at: info@nsc.org
1121 Spring Lake Drive
Itasca, IL 60143-3201
(800) 621-7615

Earthquake Country Alliance
http://www.earthquakecountry.info/dropcoverholdon/
Offers a tip sheet at:

http://www.earthquakecountry.info/downloads/ShakeOut_
Earthquake_Guide_Disabilities_AFN.pdf

Federal Emergency Management Agency (FEMA)
(800) 621-3362 (voice)
(800) 462-7585 (TTY)

Fall Prevention Center of Excellence
http://www.stopfalls.org/

National Resource Center on Supportive Housing and Home Modification
Andrus Gerontology Center
University of Southern California
3715 McClintock Avenue
Los Angeles, CA 90089-0191
(213) 740-1364 (voice)
(213) 70-7069 (fax)
homemods@usc.edu

Area Agency on Aging
Your local Area Agency on Aging provides home safety resources.

Universal Design.Com
http://www.universaldesign.com/publications/books.html

OR

Pennsylvania Housing Finance Agency
http://www.phfa.org/forms/ (Brochures, Homeownership)
Visit these sites to view and print the booklet, The Do-Able Renewable Home

Metropolitan Center for Independent Living, Inc. (MCIL)
1600 University Avenue West, Suite 16
St. Paul, MN 55104-3825
(651) 603-2029

www.wheelchairramp.org
jimwi@mcil-mn.org
Web site features "How to Build Wheelchair Ramps for Homes," an online manual for the design and construction of wheelchair ramps.

National Institute for Rehabilitation Engineering
P.O. Box T
Hewett, NJ 07421
(800) 736-2216
(973) 853-6585
nire@theoffice.net
http://www.angelfire.com/nj/nire2/

Paralyzed Veterans of America
801 18th Street NW
Washington, DC 20006-3517
(800) 424-8200 (voice)
(800) 795-HEAR (4327) (TTY)
www.pva.org
Not just for veterans, not just for paralysis. Ask for the Architecture Program.

Center for Assistive Technology and Environmental Access
Georgia Institute of Technology
490 Tenth Street, Atlanta, GA 30332-0156
http://assistivetech.net/
Their mission is to provide access to information on assistive technology (AT) devices and services, as well as on other community resources. They have a link to "what about your state" that opens to an interactive map of the U.S. for finding reuse assistive technology near you.

Check with local police to find out if they manage a **Senior Locks Program.** This program can install deadbolt locks and other security devices for homeowners 55+ who meet federal income guidelines.

Equipment and Supplies

Equipment and Supplies

*T*o provide proper at-home care, you will need certain supplies.
There are two types:

- *General medical supplies*

- *Durable medical equipment*

*Before buying anything or signing a rental contract, ask
your doctor, physical or occupational therapist, or nurse.
Salespeople may not be trained to assess what the person in
your care may need. Occupational therapists can advise you on
low-cost substitutes for expensive equipment. With the proper
doctor's orders (referrals) and documentation, some equipment
is covered by Medicare or private insurance. Get in touch with
your insurance carrier to see if what you need is covered and
follow the company's rules for getting approval before buying.*

Where to Buy Needed Supplies

Buy medical equipment and supplies from dealers that are
well established and that are well known for good service.
Be sure to get advice about where to buy from your health
care professionals or hospital discharge planner. To compare
prices, use the chart on page 151.

Look in the Yellow Pages or do an online search
under Surgical Appliances, Discount Medical Supplies,
Physicians and Surgeons, Equipment & Supplies, and First
Aid Supplies. Sources include

- Surgical supply stores

- Pharmacies or a neighborhood pharmacy store such as
  Walgreen's or CVC

- Hospitals

- Home health care agencies

- Medical supply catalogs

Where to Borrow

For short-term use, think about borrowing equipment from the following local groups:

- Salvation Army

- Red Cross

- Visiting Nurses Association

- Home health care agencies

- National Easter Seal Society

- Charity organizations

- Faith-based groups, senior centers, leisure clubs, disability focused agencies or independent living centers in your location

NOTE Never buy equipment from someone who calls you on the phone to sell you a product even if they call you by your personal name. Personal information is readily available over the Internet. Do not buy from a door- to-door salesperson.

How to Pay

If you need assistance in paying for medical equipment:

- Ask the doctor to write a prescription for a home evaluation (assessment), including an evaluation of needed equipment.

Checklist General Supplies*

- ✓ antibacterial hand cleaner (kills germs)
- ✓ bacteriostatic ointment (stops the growth of germs)
- ✓ bandages, gauze pads, tape
- ✓ blankets (2 or 3)
- ✓ cotton balls and swabs
- ✓ toothbrush, toothpaste
- ✓ denture or dental care items
- ✓ kidney-shaped basin for oral care
- ✓ container for disposing of syringes (needles)
- ✓ disposable Chux underpad that keeps moisture out, for bed protection
- ✓ draw sheets for use in turning someone in bed
- ✓ finger towels and washcloths
- ✓ foam rubber pillows
- ✓ head pillows
- ✓ heating pad
- ✓ hydrogen peroxide
- ✓ ice bag or cold pack
- ✓ hot pack or heat strips

- ✓ lotion
- ✓ 4 bed sheets (at least)
- ✓ oral laxative
- ✓ poster with first aid procedures
- ✓ pressure pad and pump
- ✓ sterile disposable gloves
- ✓ rubbing alcohol
- ✓ seat belts (to prevent sliding down in a chair)
- ✓ shower cap
- ✓ soap for dry skin
- ✓ ear thermometer
- ✓ tissues
- ✓ disposable underpants
- ✓ incontinence briefs
- ✓ panty liners
- ✓ toilet paper tongs to take care of personal hygiene
- ✓ waterproof sheeting
- ✓ roll belt restraint
- ✓ gait/transfer belt
- ✓ Medic Alert® identification

*As needed.

- If you are going through county services for in-home support ask your assessment social worker what recommended medical equipment can be paid for. You might have a waiver.

- Find out if the equipment is partly or completely covered by private health insurance with home care benefits.

- Check state retirement and union programs.

Medicare will help pay for assistive devices in some situations (wheelchairs, scooters), but does pay for durable medical equipment (home oxygen, hospital beds, walkers, wheelchairs) for home care, not in a facility. To be covered, the equipment must be prescribed by a doctor and it must be medically necessary. It must be useful only to the sick or injured person and must be reusable. Medicare will pay for the rental of certain items for no more than 15 months. After that time you may buy the equipment from the supplier or return it. If the person in your care has met the deductible, Medicare will pay 80% of the approved charges on the rental, purchase, and service of equipment that the doctor has ordered. Be aware that the amount you pay may vary because Medicare pays for different kinds of durable medical equipment in different ways.

GETTING ORGANIZED
Keep supplies together that are used often and keep a list of supplies so you can easily replace them.

Be prepared for emergencies. Have on hand a flashlight, a battery-run radio, a battery-run clock, fresh batteries, extra blankets, candles with holders, matches, and a manual can opener.

Medical Equipment

You may need to have special equipment for different rooms in the house, as well as equipment to increase the person's ability to get around.

Equipment for the Bedroom

The equipment you need to have depends on the person's medical condition. This equipment might include some of the items listed below.

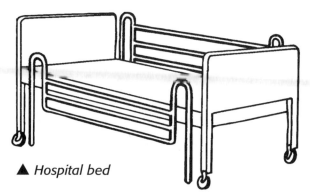

▲ *Hospital bed*

- **Hospital bed**—allows positioning (adjusting) that is not possible in a regular bed and aids in resting and breathing more comfortably and getting in and out of bed more easily

- **Alternating pressure mattress**—reduces pressure on skin tissue

- **Egg-carton pad**—a foam mattress pad shaped like the bottom of an egg carton that reduces pressure and improves air circulation

- **Portable commode chair**—for ease of toileting at the bedside

- **Trapeze bar**—provides support and a secure hand-hold while changing positions

- **Transfer board**—a smooth board for independent or assisted transfer from bed to wheelchair, toilet, or portable commode (See p. 354)

- **Hydraulic lift**—for use on a person who is difficult to move

- **Over-the-bed table**—provides a surface for eating, reading, writing, and game playing (could be an adjustable ironing board)

- **Mechanical or electric lift chair**—for help getting up from a chair

- **Blanket support**—a wire support that keeps heavy bed linens off injured areas or the feet

- **Urinal and bedpan**—for toileting in the bed

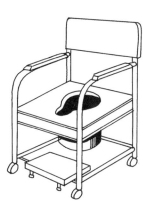

▲ *Portable commode chair*

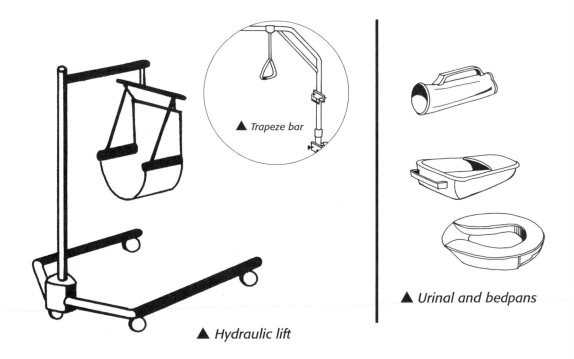

▲ *Trapeze bar*

▲ *Hydraulic lift*

▲ *Urinal and bedpans*

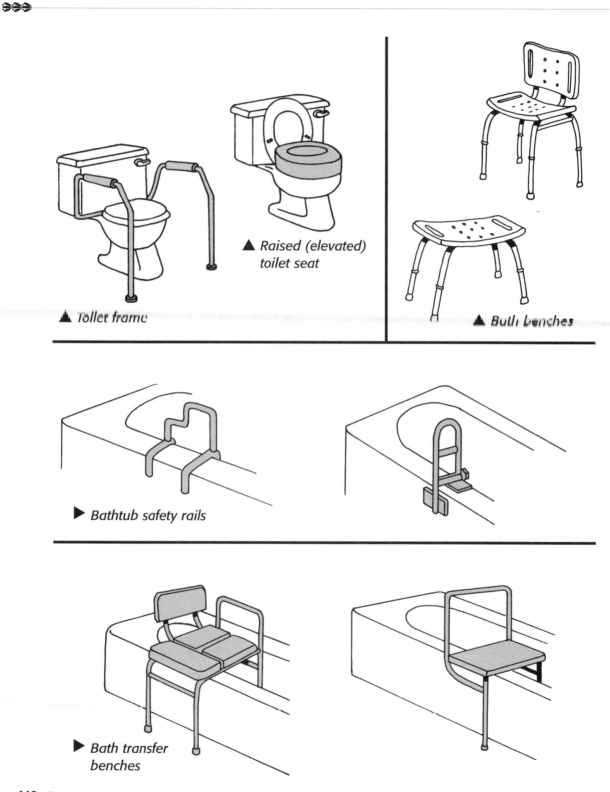

▲ Raised (elevated) toilet seat

▲ Toilet frame

▲ Bath benches

▶ Bathtub safety rails

▶ Bath transfer benches

Equipment for the Bathroom

The equipment you will need depends on the person's needs. You should consider providing the following:

- **Raised (elevated) toilet seat**—used to assist a person who has difficulty getting up or down on a toilet (available in molded plastic and clamp-on models for different toilet bowl styles)

- **Commode aid**—a device that acts as an elevated toilet seat when used with a splash guard, or as a commode when used with a pail

- **Toilet frame**—a free-standing unit that fits over the toilet and provides supports on either side for ease in getting up and down

- **Grab bars for tub and shower**—properly installed wall-mounted safety bars that hold a person's weight

- **Safety mat and strips**—rough vinyl strips that stick to the bottom of the tub and shower to prevent slipping

- **Hand-held shower hose**—a movable shower hose and head that allows the water to be directed to all parts of the body

- **Bath bench**—aid for a person who has difficulty sitting down in or getting up from the bottom of the tub

- **Bath transfer bench**—a bench that goes across the side of the tub and allows a person to get out of the tub easily

- **Bathtub safety rails**—support for getting in and out of the tub

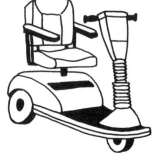

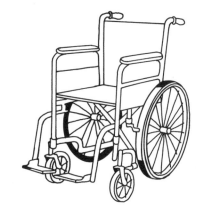

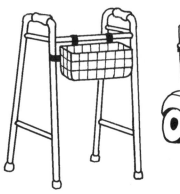

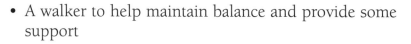

▲ Wheelchair   ▲ Walker   ▲ Electric Scooter

Mobility Aids

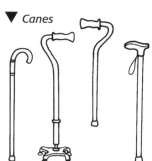

▼ Canes

Mobility aids include devices that help a person move around without help. They also help the caregiver transfer the person in and out of bed and from bed to a chair. They include—

- A wheelchair with padding and removable arms

- A walker to help maintain balance and provide some support

- A 3- or 4-wheel electric scooter

- Crutches when weight cannot be put on one leg or foot

- A cane to provide light weight-bearing support

- A transfer board (9" x 24") for moving someone in and out of bed (📖 See illustration p. 354)

- A gait/transfer belt (📖 See how to use on p. 355)

Wheelchair Requirements

Proper fit, as determined by a physical therapist.

- Safety
- Comfort
- Durability
- Ease of handling
- Ease of repair
- Cushions
- Attractive appearance

Tip

USING CANES

Choose a cane that has a wrist strap that can also be used to hang on chair or bedpost or select a cane with a hooked handle grip that easily hangs from counters or furniture. Or attach Velcro® to the top of a cane and a piece of Velcro® to counters and bedside tables to keep the cane from falling when not in use.

Wheelchair Attachments

- Brake lever extensions
- Elevated leg rests and removable footrests
- Armrests that can be taken off
- Beverage holder
- Armrest carry-all pouch to put a pad and pen or cell phone
- Tab grabber computer tablet holder
- Positioning aids to provide comfort and posture

NOTE ▷ Some states have lemon laws that cover wheelchairs and other assistive devices. If you think there is something wrong with the equipment you have bought and you want to find out if it qualifies as a "lemon," call the Attorney General's office in your state. They may be able to help you in getting a replacement or a refund.

Tip **Auto Handy Bar Transfer Aid** It is a stainless steel bar with soft, non-slip hand grip slides into car door latches to provide a strong, secure assist in getting in and out of a car. Acts as a grab bar without need for costly adaptations.

Assistive Devices

For those with poor sight and hearing or other limitations, there are many aids to make life easier. Look into all the options and you will find that your job as caregiver becomes easier too.

Sight Aids

- Prism glasses
- Magnifying glasses
- Prescription glasses
- Braille books and signs
- DVD, book recordings
- BookSense device (a portable digital audio book player accesses information for education, work, and entertainment)

- Reading machines such as Eye-Pal (a portable USB Scanner that is extremely fast and accurate. In a single keystroke it instantly converts printed material into refreshable Braille, speech or text files.)

- Augmentative and Alternative communication (AAC) devices

Listening Aids

- Hearing aids (order from an audiologist, or hearing therapist, who allows a free 30-day trial and is a registered dealer)

- Sound systems that amplify (make louder)

- Telephone amplifiers (for increased volume)

- Devices for getting close-captioned TV programs

- Doorbell sound enhancer (to make it louder) enhanced sounds and/or flashing alert light

- iPhone accessibility features

HELP FOR SPECIAL EQUIPMENT
Look into whether Medicaid or the Lion's Club in your state can pay for hearing aids.

Eating Aids

- Spoons that swivel for those who have trouble with wrist movement

- Utensils with big grip surfaces to increase the gripping so surface so they can be lifted more easily

- Plate guards or dishes with high sides that make it easier to scoop food onto a spoon

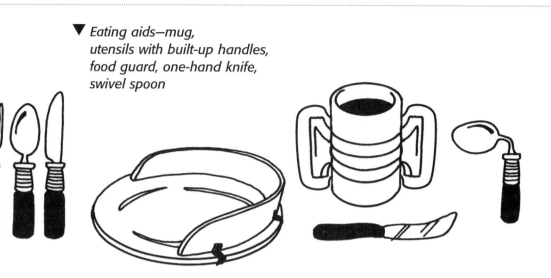

▼ *Eating aids—mug, utensils with built-up handles, food guard, one-hand knife, swivel spoon*

- Rocker knives that can cut food with a rocking motion

- Food-warming dishes for slow eaters

- Mugs with two handles, a cover, a spout, and a suction base

Dressing Aids

- Button hooks that make buttoning clothes easy

- Dressing sticks that make it possible to dress without bending

- Long-handled shoehorns so a person doesn't have to bend over when putting on shoes

- Sock aids that keep stockings open while they are being put on

- Velcro clothing that uses Velcro closures instead of buttons and zippers

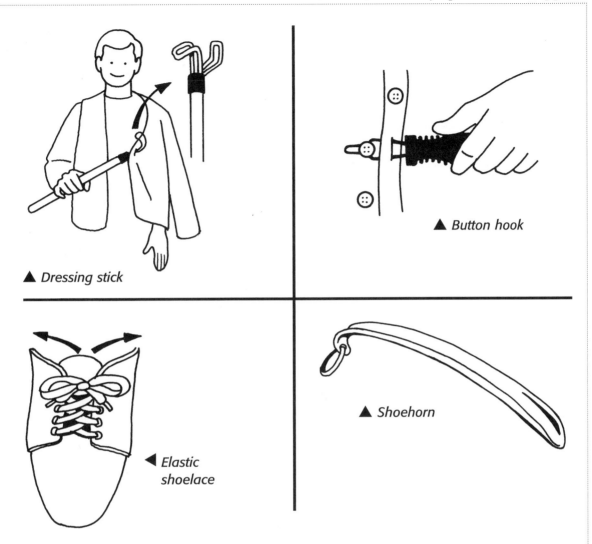

▲ *Dressing stick*

▲ *Button hook*

◀ *Elastic shoelace*

▲ *Shoehorn*

Devices for Summoning Help

- Touch-tone phones with speed dials
- Cell phone to connect with caregiver
- Medical alert response systems
- Wireless transmitters for emergency response
- iPhone monitoring and video software to stay connected

> **Tip**
>
> **Alert systems** are a good idea; at the push of a button, the system will notify a friend, caregiver, or neighbor that you need help, or call 911 or your doctor. Before shopping for an alert system, make a list of the protection features you need from an alert system. There are many alert products on the market, so it can be difficult to choose one that meets the needs of the person in your care—and is still affordable. Be wary of monthly fees or long-term contracts associated with some alert systems.
>
> Each of these products offers different features, such as range of service, medication dispensers, GPS tracking, or fall detection. See an alert system comparison at: **http://medical-alert-systems-review.toptenreviews.com/**
>
> Features to look for include 24/7 help at the push of a button, no start-up costs, no cancellation fees, no long term contracts, and low monthly costs. A system that is easy to install (for example, by plugging it into a phone line and wall receptacle using a power adapter) is a bonus. Look for free shipping, online discounts, and customer support.

Cooling Devices

Heat can be the enemy for many people with chronic illness. Learning how to "cool it!" in the summer months can be a problem. Fortunately, a number of cooling devices are available to help the caregiver and care receiver beat the heat:

- There are scarves and neck wraps that can be made cool by simply soaking in water.

- Cooling vests are another staple among cooling devices.

- Flexible non-gel cold pads that contour to the body.

- There are devices for cooling wrists and ankles. One brand has arm and leg bands made of terrycloth into which you insert custom-size freezer packs.

- Cooling fans. Check with your community senior centers or elder care locations; many they collect fan donations to give to seniors during hot months.

Computer Equipment

Countless hardware and software programs can make computers easier to use for people with disabilities. Alternative keyboards, puff switches for those who cannot use a mouse, screen readers, talking word processors, and voice recognition software like **Dragon NaturallySpeaking** are available today. Talk to an occupational therapist or with one of the salespeople at a computer or electronics store for ideas on making computers more accessible.

Homemade Aids and Gadgets

- Wrist straps for canes—tape tied on a cane so it can be hung from the wrist while walking upstairs

- Bicycle baskets—strapped to a walker to store necessities and leave the hands free

- An egg carton—to organize pills

- Rubber safety mats—ideal for the tub, shower, or any slippery surface; also useful to make place on trays and tables for a nonslip surface

- Key—put the end of the key that you hold into a large cork for ease of grip

- Foot-operated door levers—made by attaching rope to a "stirrup" and tying it to the lever handle

- Language tags—cardboard tags with words that can be used to express needs

- Light-switch enlargements—made by putting a rubber pen cap over a light switch

- Enlarged pull switches—made by putting a plastic ball over small switches

- Clips for canes—spring clips or Velcro® placed on favorite chairs to keep a cane from falling

- Bedside rails—wooden rails attached to the floor at right angles on swivel hinges

- Pull rope—rope attached to the footboard of the bed to help someone change positions in bed

Specialized Hospital-Type Equipment

- **Oxygen tanks**, for use when oxygen is needed as a medication

- **Breathing tube (transtracheal oxygen therapy equipment)**, for use when oxygen is delivered into the lungs through a flexible tube that goes from the neck directly into the trachea (sometimes called the windpipe)

- **Compressors and hand-held nebulizers (inhalers)**, which reduce medication to a form that can be inhaled

- **Suction catheters**, which clear mucus and secretions from the back of the throat when someone cannot swallow

- **Home infusion equipment**, or IV (intravenous) therapy, which delivers antibiotics, blood products, chemotherapy, hydration (water), pain management, parenteral (IV) nutrition, and specialty medications

Equipment Cost-Comparison Chart (Example)

Item	Purchase Price	Rental Fee × Months Needed	Covered by Medicare Yes/No	Vendor
bath stool	$			
bedpan				
bed safety				
accessories				
cane				
commode				
crutches				
hospital bed				
mattress				
oxygen				
raised toilet seat				
special equipment				
trapeze				
walker				
wheelchair				
3-or 4-wheel scooter				
other				
Totals	$			

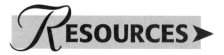

RESOURCES ➤

To find a supplier who is enrolled in the Medicare program, visit
www.medicare.gov and select "Find Suppliers of Medical Equipment in Your Area." You can also call (800) MEDICARE (800-633-4227) for this information. TTY users should call (877) 486-2048.

Caregiver Products (daily living aids)
(877) 750-0376 M–F, 8 a.m.–5 p.m. (CST)
http://www.caregiverproducts.com/
Shop for in home care, stroke, elderly, Parkinson's, disabled, handicapped, and geriatric caregiver aids, products, and supplies.

Adaptive Technology Resources
(262) 375-2020 (local)
(800) 770-8474 (toll free)
(262) 375-6777 (fax)
http://www.adaptivetr.com/

American Speech-Language-Hearing Association
(800) 638-8255 (non-members)
(301) 296-8580 (fax)
(301) 296-5650 (TTY)
http://www.asha.org

AbilityHub Assistive Technology Solutions
(802) 775-1993
(802) 773-1604 (fax)
info@abilityhub.com
http://abilityhub.com/index.htm
Assistive technology for people who have difficulty operating a computer

ABLEDATA
(800) 227-0216
(301) 608-8998 (voice)
(301) 608-8912 (TTY)
(301) 608-8958 (fax)
abledata@macrointernational.com
www.abledata.com
Stores information on thousands of assistive devices for home health care, from eating utensils to wheelchairs. Provides prices, names, and addresses of suppliers.

Institute for Human Centered Design (formerly Adaptive Environments)
(617) 695-1225 (v/TTY)
(617) 482-8099 (fax)
info@HumanCenteredDesign.org

Alliance for Technology Access
(800) 914-3017
(731) 554-5282 (voice)
(731) 554-5284 (TTY)
(731) 554-5283 (fax)
atainfo@ataccess.org
www.ataccess.org
A network of community-based resource centers, developers, vendors, and associates dedicated to providing information and support services to children and adults with disabilities and increasing their use of standard, assistive, and information technologies.

American Occupational Therapy Association (AOTA)
(301) 652-2682 (voice)
(800) 377-8555 (TDD)
(301) 652-7711 (fax)
www.aota.org
Provides consumer publications.

Apple Computer Accessibility

accessibility@apple.com
www.apple.com/accessibility
Committed to helping people with disabilities to access their computers. Apple computer operating systems are considered best when a cognitive impairment or loss of short-term memory is present.

AT&T Special Needs Center

(877) 902-6350 (voice)
(800) 772-2889 (TTY)
Provides free directory assistance (with an application) and operator's help with dialing for those who are vision impaired or disabled.

Briggs Healthcare

(800) 247-2343
(800) 222-1996 (fax)
www.briggscorp.com

Independent Living Research Utilization at TIRR

(713) 520-0232 (voice/TTY)
(713) 520-5785 (fax)
ilru@ilru.org, www.ilru.org

Lighthouse International

(800) 829-0500
(212) 821-9200
info@lighthouse.org
www.lighthouse.org
Provides free information on eye-related diseases and can refer individuals to resources in your community. Online store of low-vision aides. Includes numerous tip sheets and publications; features a "Help Near You" function to find resources in your area.

Microsoft Accessibility Technology for Everyone

www.microsoft.com/enable
A Web site of products, training, and free resources to make technology accessible to everyone.

National Rehabilitation Information Center for Independence

(800) 346-2742 (voice)
(301) 459-5984 (TTY)
(301) 459-4263 (fax)
naricinfo@heitechservices.com
www.naric.com
A database of research information about assistive technology and rehabilitation. One-stop shopping for referrals, information, and equipment sources. Fees for some services.

North Coast Medical Rehabilitation Catalog

www.ncmedical.com
(800) 821-9319

Radio Shack

Carries a variety of alerting devices in stores nationwide. Check your local store or search online.

Sammons-Preston

(630) 378-6000
(630) 378-6010 (fax)
sp@pattersonmedical.com

Sears Health and Wellness Catalogue

http://www.sears.com/
(800) 697-3277 for customer service
Call to place an order or find a Sears store near you. Sears may install air conditioners or heaters at no charge if these are medically needed and income qualifying.

Hearing Loss Association of America

(301) 657-2248
Offers information on coping with hearing loss and on hearing aids.

SpeciaLiving Magazine
www.specialiving.com
Online info and store for accessible housing, special products, such as ramps, bathing systems, urinary devices, lifts.

World Institute on Disability
(510) 225-6400 (TTY)
(510) 225-0478
(510) 225-0477 (fax)
wid@wid.org
www.wid.org

Publication

Warner, Mark L. Warner, Ellen. *The Complete Guide to Alzheimer's Proofing Your Home*. West Lafayette, Indiana. Purdue University Press. 2000.
This extremely useful guide deals with both interior and exterior spaces and shows how to create a home environment for people with Alzheimer's and related dementias. The book provides an exhaustive directory of manufacturers to locate the latest products for home health care.

At Download Provider, *The Complete Guide to Alzheimer's Proofing Your Home*. Mark Warner and Ellen Warner. Revised downloadable edition 2013, http://www.downloadprovider. me/en/

For **medical alarms**, go online at: http://medical-alert-systems-review.toptenreviews.com/ to compare systems, or consult the phone book or contact your local hospital's long-term care or senior services division

If you don't have access to the Internet, ask your local library or senior center to help you locate a Web site.

Part Two: Day by Day

Part 2

Day by Day

Setting Up a Plan of Care

Setting Up a Plan of Care

A plan of care is a daily record of the care and treatment a person needs after a hospital stay. The plan helps you and the person in your care with caregiving tasks.

When a person leaves a hospital, the discharge planner provides the caregiver with a copy of the doctor's orders and a brief set of instructions for care. The discharge planner also works with a home health care agency to send a nurse, The nurse will evaluate the patient's needs for equipment, personal care, help with shots or medication, etc. The nurse will also work with the entire health care team (including you as the caregiver, a physical therapist, and other specialists) to develop a detailed plan of care.

The plan of care includes the following information:

- Diagnosis (the nature of the disease)

- Medications

- Functional limitations (what the person can and cannot do)

- A list of equipment needed

- Special diet

- Detailed care instructions and comments

- Services the home health care agency provides

The information is presented in a certain order so that the process of care is repeated over and over until it becomes routine. When the plan is kept up to date, it provides a clear record of events that helps solve problems and avoid them.

With a plan, you don't have to rely on your memory. It also allows another person to take over respite care or take your place entirely without too much trouble.

Some of the things you may have to watch and record are

- Skin color, warmth, and tone (dryness, firmness, etc.)

- Pressure areas where bedsores can develop (📖 see **Activities of Daily Living**, p. 228)

- Breathing, temperature, pulse, and blood pressure

- Circulation (dark red or blue spots on the legs or feet)

- Fingernails and toenails (any unusual conditions)

- Mobility (ability to move around)

- Puffiness around the eyes and cheeks, swelling of the hands and ankles

- Appetite

- Body posture (relaxed, twisted, or stiff)

- Bowel and bladder function (unusual changes)

Recording the Plan of Care

Use a loose-leaf notebook to record the plan of care. Put the doctor's instructions on the inside front cover (always keep the originals). Include in the notebook the types of forms that appear in the following pages of this chapter. These pages should be three-hole punched.

After using your plan of care for one week, make changes as needed and continue to do so as the person's needs change. Always do what works for you and the person in your care. Use notes, pictures, or anything else to describe your responsibilities. Also, use black ink, not pencil, to keep a permanent record.

Daily Activities Record (Sample Form)   Day/Date: _____

Morning _____

_____

Afternoon _____

Naps: Time _____ Place _____

Evening _____

Activities	Yes	No	Where/How/When
Walk	❏	❏	_____
TV	❏	❏	_____
Reading Aloud	❏	❏	_____
Visitors	❏	❏	_____
Calls to Friends/Relatives	❏	❏	_____
Other _____			_____

Bedtime Routine	Yes	No	Where/How
Incontinence Pad/Brief	❏	❏	_____
Medication	❏	❏	_____
Special Pillow/Blanket	❏	❏	_____
Music/Radio/TV	❏	❏	_____
Nightlight	❏	❏	_____
Restraints, Calming Techniques	❏	❏	_____
Urinal/Bedpan	❏	❏	_____
Gates at Doors/on Stairs	❏	❏	_____
Oral/Denture Care	❏	❏	_____
Foot Care	❏	❏	_____

Braces ❏   Fungus ❏   Massage ❏   Ingrown Nails ❏   Nail Care ❏

Meals

Help Needed with Meals _____

Meal Times _____

Special Diet _____

Foods to Avoid _____

Special Utensils _____

Snacks _____

Favorite Foods _____

Location of Meals _____

Daily Care Record (Sample Form)   Day/Date: _____

Daily Activities/Limitations:

Walks Alone _____ Stands Alone _____

Bed Position _____

Equipment Used: Walker ❏   Cane ❏   Wheelchair ❏   Brace ❏

How long _____

ROM/Exercises: Upper Body ❏   Lower Body ❏   Goes Outside ❏

Meals: Special Diet   ❏

Breakfast _____

Lunch _____

Dinner _____

Snack _____

Fluids _____

Treatments

Catheter _____

Oxygen _____

Equipment _____

Physical Therapy _____

Special Precautions _____

Resuscitate ❏   **Do Not Resuscitate ❏**

Personal Care

Bath: ❏ Bed   ❏ Chair

Shower: ❏ Tub   ❏ Bench

Care of Genitals: _____

Nail Care: ❏ Toes   ❏ Fingers

Oral Care: ❏ Brush Teeth   ❏ Floss Teeth   ❏ Dentures

Hair Care: ❏ Shave   ❏ Bed Shampoo   ❏ Bath/Shampoo

Skin Care: ❏ Lotion Upper Body   ❏ Lotion Lower Body   ❏ Powdered

Massage: ❏ Head and Shoulder   ❏ Leg and Foot   ❏ Back

Bowel Movements _____ Voiding _____ Quantity _____

Temperature _____ Blood Pressure _____ Respiration _____

Comments/Attitudes/Conditions _____

_____

_____

Visitors _____

Activities Schedule for Backup Caregiver (Sample Form)

Personal Needs	Yes	No	Where to Find
Cane	❏	❏	_____
Dentures	❏	❏	_____
Glasses	❏	❏	_____
Hearing aid	❏	❏	_____
Walker	❏	❏	_____

Morning Routine

Breakfast _____ Where Eaten _____

Amount of Help Needed _____

Special Utensils Needed _____

Medications with Meals ❏ _____ Nap ❏ _____

Snack Foods _____ Time of Snack _____

Evening Routine

Dinner _____ Where Eaten _____

Evening Snack _____

Bedtime Routine

Help Needed Undressing ❏ _____ Shower or Bath Needed ❏ _____

Where Clothes Are Stored _____

Where Dentures Are Stored _____

Special Items Needed: _____

Incontinent Pad/Brief ❏ _____ Urinal ❏ _____ Restraints ❏ _____

Special Pillows ❏ _____ Music ❏ _____ Nightlight ❏ _____

Calming Techniques _____

_____

Special Concerns or Equipment

Catheter ❏ _____ Oxygen ❏ _____

Special Precautions _____

Other _____

Resuscitate ❏   **Do Not Resuscitate ❏**

Be on the Alert for:

Gates on Stairs/Locks on Doors _____

Alarms _____

Other _____

Don't be surprised if: _____

Recording and Managing Medications

Always be sure that the person in your care takes the medication exactly as prescribed. Keep an accurate list of these medications and when they should be taken.

Never make any changes to these medications without talking to the doctor or specialist first. However, because everyone's treatment needs are different, the specialist may want to try changing the amount or timing of drugs, within certain limits. If you are worried or have any questions, don't be afraid to ask your doctor or pharmacist for advice.

People who have serious health problems often take a large number of medications at many different times of the day. It is essential to have a careful system for keeping track of medications:

- When medications should be given

- How they should be given

- When they were actually given

The following sample of a weekly medication schedule is a good model to follow. Be sure to fill in the times when (A.M. and P.M.) medications actually were given, and have each caregiver initial them.

Weekly Medication Schedule (Sample Form)

Medication	Date/Time/Initials						
Name, dose, frequency, with or without food	Sat.	Sun.	Mon.	Tues.	Wed.	Thurs.	Fri.
Example							
Coumadin 2mg 1x daily a.m. with food							
Folic acid 400mg 1x daily a.m.							
Vitamin/mineral capsule 1x daily, with food • Noon							
Artificial tears 2x daily • 8 a.m. • bedtime							

As you finish your own schedule, be sure to record information from the label of each prescription, including

- Days of the week when each medicine must be taken

- Number of times per day

- Time of day

- Whether the medicine is to be taken with or without food

- How much water should be taken with the medicine

Also make a note to yourself about any warnings (for example, "Don't take this medicine with alcohol") and possible side effects (dizziness, confusion, headache, etc.).

> **NOTE** 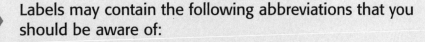 Labels may contain the following abbreviations that you should be aware of:
>
> **HS**—hour of sleep (medication time)
> **BID**—give the medicine 2 times per day (approximately 8AM and 8PM)
> **TID**—give the medicine 3 times per day (approximately 9AM, 1PM, 6PM)
> **QID**—give the medicine 4 times per day (approximately 9AM, 1PM, 5PM, 9PM)

Other Cautions

- Never crush drugs without talking to the doctor or pharmacist first. If the person in your care has trouble swallowing medication, ask the doctor if there is another way it can be taken. (📖 See ***Using the Health Care Team Effectively***, p. 35)

- If the person in your care will take the medicine without your help, ask the pharmacist to use easy-open caps on prescription bottles.

- Do not store medicine that will be taken internally (swallowed) in the same cabinet with medicine that will be used externally (lotions, salves, creams, etc.).

- Keep a magnifying glass near the medicine cabinet for reading small print.

- Store most medicine in a cool, dry place—usually not the bathroom.

- Remove the cotton from each bottle so that moisture is not drawn in.

- Flush all medicine not currently being used down the toilet.

- If childproof containers are too hard to open, ask the pharmacist for containers that are not childproof.

Tip

EMERGENCY PREPAREDNESS
Let the local fire station and ambulance company know that a person with disabilities lives at your address. They will have the information on hand and can respond quickly.

Your Notes

Emergency Information

Have this information posted near telephones or on the refrigerator, where it can be used by anyone in the household in case of emergency.

Personal Information

Name _____ Date of Birth _____

Address _____

Phone _____

SS # _____ Supplemental Insurance # _____

Medicaid # _____ Medicare # _____

Current Medications: _____

_____

Exact Location of Do Not Resuscitate Order: _____

Emergency Numbers

Fire _____ Police _____

Ambulance _____ Hospital _____

Doctor _____

Drugstore _____ Open Till _____ Delivers _____

Family Caregiver Work Number _____

Alternate Caregiver _____

Home Health Care Agency _____

Medicare Toll Free Number _____

Insurance _____

Medical Equipment Company _____

Poison Control _____

Friend _____

_____

Neighbor _____ Relative _____

Clergy/Rabbi _____

Transport Number _____ Meals-on-Wheels _____

Shopping Assistance _____

Directions for Driving to the House _____

_____

_____

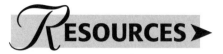

RESOURCES ➤

United Hospital Fund's Next Step In Care Campaign
www.nextstepincare.org
The Centers for Medicare and Medicaid Services (CMS) and the United Hospital Fund's Next Step in Care campaign collaborated on a series of six podcasts called "**Helping Patients & Family Caregivers Take the Next Step in Care: Medication Management.**"

General Caregiving Books

Always on Call: When Illness Turns Families into Caregivers, by Carol Levine (Ed.), New York. United Hospital Fund, 2000.

The Complete Eldercare Planner, by Joy Loverde, Pittsburgh, PA. Three Rivers Press, 2000.

Taking Care of Aging Family Members, by Wendy Lustbader, New York. Free Press, 1994.

If you don't have home access to the Internet, ask your local library to help you locate any Web site.

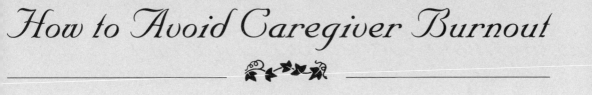

How to Avoid Caregiver Burnout

How to Avoid Caregiver Burnout

*P*roviding emotional support and physical care to an ill person can be deeply satisfying, but it can be upsetting. Sometimes it is simply more than one person can handle. The strain of balancing a job, a family, more work in the home, and the care of someone may lead you to feel resentful or angry and guilty.

One of the biggest mistakes caregivers make is thinking that they can—and should—do everything by themselves. The best way to avoid burnout is to have the practical and emotional support of other people. Sharing concerns with others not only relieves stress, but also can give you a new slant on problems.

Negative Emotions That May Arise in You

The challenges of the caregiver role may sometimes make you feel bad about yourself. If you are a perfectionist, you'll never do it perfectly. If you're angry, you'll find plenty of excuses to be mad. If you have feelings of inadequacy, they'll definitely come up. Impatience, depression, hostility—even if these emotions did not challenge you before, they're sure to arise in this situation. The job is a challenging one, and it can be life changing.

Guilt Is Crippling

Opportunities for guilt can come up often in caregiving. Even if you are doing everything right, you can easily convince yourself that you're not doing enough. To combat this tendency, *at least once a day, every day*, remind yourself:

- About how you are helping the person in your care

- When you don't do everything needed in a day, you are doing what you can with love

- You have grown in skill and compassion, learning on the job

Depression Is Dangerous

Just as depression endangers your care receiver's recovery, it also endangers your health and well-being. Depression increases your risk in every major disease category, particularly cardiovascular disease.

Symptoms of Depression

Here are the symptoms:

- Persistent sad, anxious or "empty" mood

- Feelings of hopelessness, pessimism

- Feelings of guilt, worthlessness, helplessness

- Loss of interest or pleasure in hobbies and activities that were once enjoyed, including sex

- Decreased energy, fatigue, being "slowed down"

- Difficulty concentrating, remembering, making decisions

- Insomnia, early-morning awakening, or oversleeping

- Appetite and/or weight changes

- Thoughts of death or suicide, or suicidal attempts

- Restlessness, irritability

- Substance abuse

If you have five or more of these symptoms for longer than two weeks, depression may be the cause. Talk to a physician, psychiatrist, or psychologist about treatment options. The effective treatment might be to combine medication with talking therapy.

- Claim time for yourself and make sure you use it; otherwise, you will burn out and the person in your care will suffer.

- Make and keep doctor's appointments for yourself; otherwise, when you get sick, everyone will suffer.

- Join a caregiver support group; otherwise, you and the person in your care may suffer isolation.

- Take advantage of respite care opportunities, otherwise, when you break down the person in your care will suffer.

 Tip A caregiver support group offers a place to gain practical information on local resources, like who to talk with at agencies that were helpful to others in your group

Anger

It is easy to feel victimized in this situation; you are caught up in someone else's illness. The natural response is anger. Unfortunately, that is not a helpful response. Unleashing anger on the person in your care never helps.

On the other hand, it is not good for you to stuff those feelings. There are definite consequences to your health and well-being. Try these outlets:

- Caregiver support groups provide a place where you can vent feelings. Everyone there understands; no one will make you feel guilty. Members will often offer effective, real-world solutions. Scientific evidence indicates caregivers who participate in support groups are better able to deal with the situation.

- Make an appointment with a therapist or family counselor or clergyperson. If possible, make two appointments: one for you alone and one for you and the person in your care.

- Keep a journal of your feelings.

- Remember, people who have lost control may try to regain it by controlling what they can, which may be their caregivers.

- Separate the person from the condition. The illness, not the person in your care, is responsible for the difficulties and challenges that you both are facing. Don't blame the care receiver for the situation you are in.

- Set and enforce limits on how many non-essential needs you will fill per hour, such as pouring water or changing channels. Non-emergency care does not have to be handled immediately.

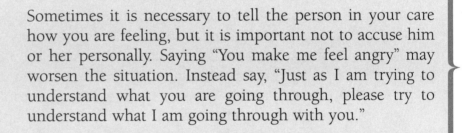

Tip

Sometimes it is necessary to tell the person in your care how you are feeling, but it is important not to accuse him or her personally. Saying "You make me feel angry" may worsen the situation. Instead say, "Just as I am trying to understand what you are going through, please try to understand what I am going through with you."

Emotional Burdens

You may think you are the only one to face these problems, but you are not alone. Every caregiver faces—

- The need to hide his or her grief

- Fear of the future

- Worries about money

- Having less ability to solve problems

- Grieving the loss of independence and your social
  network

Dependency and Isolation

Fears of dependency and loneliness, or isolation, are common
in families of those who are ill. The person needing care
can become more and more dependent on the one who is
providing it. At the same time, the caregiver needs others
for respite and support. Many caregivers are ashamed about
needing help, so they don't ask for it. Those caregivers who
are able to develop personal and social support have a greater
sense of well-being.

Knowing When to Seek Help

"Why doesn't anyone ask how I am doing?" It is easy to
feel invisible, as if no one can see you. Everyone's attention
is on the person with the illness, and they don't seem to
understand what the caregiver is going through. Many
caregivers say that nobody even asks how they're doing.
Mental health experts say it's not wise to let feelings of
neglect build up. Caregivers need to speak up and tell other
people what they need and how they feel.

Support groups, religious or spiritual advisors, or mental
health counselors can teach you new and positive ways to
express your own need for help.

Seek out professional help when you:

- Are using more alcohol than usual to cope

- Are using too many prescription medications

- Have physical symptoms such as skin rashes, backaches,
  or a cold or flu that won't go away

- Are unable to think clearly or focus

- Feel tired and don't want to do anything

- Feel keyed up and on edge

- Feel sad all the time

- Feel intense fear and anxiety

- Feel worthless

- Are depressed for two weeks or more

- Are having thoughts of suicide

- Have become or are thinking about becoming physically violent toward the person you are caring for

When Hostility Builds to the Breaking Point

Anger is a common emotion for caregivers and for the person being cared for. The situation feels—and is—unfair. Both may say hurtful words during a difficult task. Someone may slam a door during a disagreement. Shouting sometimes replaces conversation. Anger and frustration must be addressed and healthy outlets found as a way to let off steam. If they are not, angry situations can become physically or emotionally abusive. (📖 See ***Abuse***, p. 265). You can control your emotions by letting go of anger and frustration in a safe way.

- Take a walk to cool down.

- Write your thoughts in a journal.

- Go to a private corner and take out your anger on a big pillow.

- Claim a caregiver hour each day. Pick a favorite time or spot and declare it your time.

Checklist **Dealing with Physical and Emotional Burdens**

✓ Do not allow the person in your care to take unfair advantage of you by being overly demanding.

✓ Live one day at a time.

✓ List priorities, decide what to leave undone, and think of ways to make the work easier.

✓ When doing a long, boring care task, use the time to relax or listen to music.

✓ Find time for regular exercise to increase your energy (even if you only stretch in place).

✓ Focus on getting relaxing sleep rather than more sleep.

✓ Take several short rests in order to get enough sleep.

✓ Set aside time for prayer or personal reflection.

✓ Practice deep breathing and learn to meditate to empty your mind of all troubles.

✓ Allow your self-esteem to rise because you have discovered hidden skills and talents.

✓ Realize your own limitations and accept them.

✓ Make sure your goals are realistic—you may be unable to do everything you could do before.

✓ Keep your eating habits balanced—do not fall into a toast-and-tea habit.

✓ Take time for yourself.

✓ Treat yourself to a massage.

✓ Keep up with outside friends and activities.

✓ Spread the word that you would welcome some help, and allow friends and family to help with respite care.

✓ Delegate (assign) jobs to others. Keep a list of tasks you need to have done and assign specific ones when people offer to help. (See resources section for online calendar help.)

✓ Share your concerns with a friend.

✓ Join a support group, or start one (to share ideas and resources).

✓ Use respite care when needed.

✓ Express yourself openly and honestly with people you feel should be doing more to help.

✓ When you visit your own doctor, be sure to explain your caregiving responsibilities, not just your symptoms.

✓ Allow yourself to feel your emotions without guilt. They are natural and very human.

✓ Unload your anger and frustration by writing it down.

✓ Allow yourself to cry and sob.

✓ Know that you are providing a very important service to the person in your care.

Where to Find Professional Help or Support Groups

- The community pages of the phone directory or online
- The local county medical society, which can provide a list of counselors, psychologists, and psychiatrists
- Religious service agencies
- Community health clinics
- Religious and spiritual advisors
- United Way's 24/7 dial 211 or (800) 543-7709
- If the person in your care has recently been discharged from a health care facility, contact the hospital's discharge planner (social worker)
- A newspaper calendar listing of support group meetings
- Parish nurses
- Area Agency on Aging
- Ask for help from a counselor who is familiar with the needs of caregivers.
- Online discussion groups or phone support 24/7 from the Alzheimer's Association

Self-Care for Caregivers

If you don't take care of yourself, then you won't finish the caregiving race, and the care receiver will suffer. Part of your responsibility to the person in your care is to take care of yourself.

> *Tip* Here's a thought to keep in mind: Before every flight, during the safety talk given by the flight attendants, they tell parents that, in case of trouble, to put the oxygen mask on themselves first and then on the child. Why? Because if the parent passes out the child's safety is at risk.

Exercise

Even moderate exercise is beneficial because it breaks the cycle of being sedentary. And being sedentary is a risk factor for all major diseases.

Walking is easy, and if you can't walk for 30–40 minutes at a stretch, several 5–10 minute periods are enough. Exercise improves mood and physique and can be an opportunity to socialize. Find a way to make it part of your day.

> *Tip* If you can't join a gym, investigate the YMCA. Some larger churches often have low-or no-cost exercise classes. Community pools often have low-cost adult swim and exercise classes. Local yoga or Tai Chi classes can be offered on a sliding scale as with community recreation programs.

Eat Right

Nutrition is critical to your well-being. Learn to read labels and avoid foods with high fat content. Vary your protein food choices. Twice a week, make seafood the protein on your plate. Eat beans, which are a natural source of fiber and protein. Keep meat and poultry portions small and lean—learn more at: **www.FoodSafety.gov**.

The person in your care will almost certainly be given a dietary prescription. In cooking heart-healthy for him, you will benefit yourself and the rest of your family as well.

Drink plenty of water and avoid sugary drinks and sodium. (📖 See **Diet, Nutrition, and Exercise**, p. 283)

Tip

Do you know there are about 10 packets of sugar in a 12-ounce can of soda? A recent Purdue University study (July 2013) "found that diet soda drinkers who maintained a healthy weight range *still* had a significantly increased risk of the top three killers in the United States: diabetes, heart disease and stroke."

Calorie-dense foods pack a lot of calories in a small package—think chocolate. For example, 8 oz of broccoli is 65 calories; 8 oz of chocolate chip cookies is 1,070 calories. Fresh fruits and vegetables will typically have many fewer calories than processed foods and be filling. Canned fruit often has added sugar; canned vegetables generally have added salt.

Tip

Most people need to eat more fruit—2 cups a day. To help you meet that goal, keep a bowl of apples, oranges, pears, bananas, and seasonal fruits on the kitchen counter and nibble on fruit throughout the day. Your veggie intake should be around 3 to 4½ cups each day.

Tip

For reliable and easy-to-understand information on nutrition; changing your diet; easy-to-follow eating plans; and quick, tasty, and healthy recipes, visit **www.AmericanHeart.org**. It is a free, one-stop shop for heart-healthy nutrition.

Take Care of the Caregiver

Many caregivers neglect their own physical health. They ignore what is ailing them and don't take steps to avoid getting sick, such as exercising, eating a proper diet, and getting regular medical examinations.

Many caregivers do not get enough sleep at night. If sleep is regularly broken up because the person in your care needs help during the night, talk about the problems with a health care professional.

The person in your care needs a healthy caregiver. Both partners need uninterrupted sleep.

Meditation

Your journey as a caregiver could be more satisfying and less stressful if you take up a practice of daily meditation. Think of meditation as sitting still doing nothing. Here are seven easy steps:

1. Sit so your back is straight, either on a chair or a big, firm pillow.

2. As you inhale, tense your whole body—arms, legs, buttocks, fists, scrunch your face.

3. Hold 2–3 seconds.

4. Exhale and relax (repeat twice).

5. Take a deep breath, let your belly expand.

6. Exhale and relax (repeat twice).

7. Breathe normally and observe your thoughts for five minutes.

> **Tip**
>
> Most people fail at meditation because they think meditation means clearing your mind of thoughts. Instead of emptying your mind of thoughts, observe them. There are no "right" thoughts to think. Don't focus on any of your thoughts and don't fight with any of them. An easy way to do that is to label each one as it bubbles up—sad thought, happy thought, angry thought, depressed thought, to-do list thought—and let it go. Then label the next one that appears. The goal remains the same: to achieve positive thinking for better overall health.

> **Tip**
>
> A kitchen timer will alert you when your five minutes are up. So can your smartphone, using either the calendars option or the phone's stopwatch or counter.

It is not important how long you sit with your eyes closed and observe your thoughts—5 minutes will do, especially to start. What makes meditation effective at reducing stress is the practice of meditation, doing it every day. You can do it before the person in your care wakes up or after she goes to bed or is taking a nap. It's only 5 or 10 minutes, but the cumulative effect over just a few weeks is noticeable.

Plan for the Long Term: Winning the Caregiving Race

Most people jump into caregiving as if it were a sprint. They think they can and must do everything themselves. You may be able to do that for a few weeks or even months, but the average caregiver spends more than four years in that role—no one can sprint for that long.

Instead of a sprint, treat caregiving as a marathon— for which you have not trained—and pace yourself accordingly from the start. Find effective ways to share or get help from others.

Tip

If you find yourself in an angry conversation with the person in your care *in your head,* **get it out in the open.**
- Find a counselor or therapist to talk to.
- Talk to a neutral third party, even if it's by phone or e-mail.
- Tap into a local or online support group.
- Keep a journal.

Respite Time

Every caregiver needs respite time if she is to last. It may be hard to think of yourself and your needs at this time, but if you don't, your life will be consumed by your duties and you will burn out. Respite (a temporary break from responsibility) is not a luxury, it is a necessity.

Your care receiver's level of disability determines whether he or she can be left alone and for how long. Care options include—

- Asking a family member or friend to stay with your care receiver for an hour or two

- Taking him or her to adult daycare (if eligible; most programs have transport to and from the program if the care receiver can get to the sidewalk for pickup/drop off).

- Employing a professional sitter or health care aide for a few hours a week or month

- Hiring a college student (if skilled care is not needed) to stay with your care receiver for a while several times a week

- Enrolling the person in your care in a support group

Check with your local Area Agency on Aging, ARCH, or Easter Seals for respite-care programs in your area. Larger churches often have outreach programs that include respite care.

However you are able to arrange for some help—and it will take some effort on your part, it won't happen by itself—commit to taking some time at least once a week to do something for yourself.

NOTE To make this happen you will have to defend this time because other things will demand to be made a priority. If you do not defend your respite time, you will not get it or the renewal it generates. Remember, caregiving is a marathon, not a sprint—respite time helps you finish the race.

Respite Zone

A respite zone is an area within your home set aside just for you, the caregiver. The idea is that this is your space. It can be your bedroom, the spare room, an office, or even a bench outside in the garden or on a porch. This is a place for you to take a break while the person in your care rests or is taken care of by someone else.

In creating your respite zone,

- Keep in mind what you want to do there. Reading? Painting? Writing? Gardening? Bubble bath? Surf the web? Music?

- Identify the time you will use as respite—during nap time, when someone relieves you? If you can only get a break at night after the person in your care is in bed, gardening probably won't do, but watching a movie or favorite TV show might.

- Identify free space in your home—porches are good candidates, a spare room is perfect, maybe a corner of your bedroom. A screen can give you privacy if you can't close the door.

- Modify the space according to your needs—a reading chair with a lamp or a stereo headset. Keep whatever is necessary for your respite activity. Or get a mobile laptop computer.

Your respite zone should be your creation alone. The goal is to give you a place of your own where you can find enjoyment in your own home and life. If searching the Internet is fun for you, your zone will be different from someone who wants to take a bubble bath and listen to soft music. Creative projects such as painting, sewing, writing, baking, gardening, and photography are excellent ways to absorb your attention and take your mind off your responsibilities.

Your respite zone should be just for you. You need to feel secure that your things are safe and will not be disturbed or discarded. It is important for your care receiver to understand that this space is yours.

> *Tip*
>
> It is not selfish to set aside space and time for yourself, because if you fail to give yourself space, time, and the opportunity to be with your own thoughts, your caregiving journey will be harder on you than it has to be.

Taking care of a debilitated (weakened) family member or friend who may not recover completely can be an all-consuming job. However, if you allow it to consume all of you because you do not demand some time and space for yourself, what will happen to the person in your care when you collapse?

Respite care is not a luxury. It is necessary for the well-being of the person in your care and for you.

Changes in Attitude Relieve Stress

Here are some suggestions to help reduce your stress level:

- Learn to say no. Good boundaries improve relationships and provide needed structure

- Control your attitude: Don't dwell on what you lack or what you can't change.

- Appreciate what you have and can do.

- Go on a TV diet. Find simple ways to have fun: Play a board game, organize family photos, listen to music you enjoy, read the biography of an inspiring person.

- Learn a time-management tool, like making a to-do list (specifically include items that you enjoy).

- Knowledge is empowering; get information about your care receiver's condition.

- Find a support system and nurture it.

- Share your feelings with someone who will listen.

- Keep a gratitude journal—record three new things you are grateful for every day.

- Memorize an inspiring poem.

- Tune into BlogTalk online radio programs for caregiver, senior, or support programming for disabilities

The #1 thing you can do to improve your situation is to acknowledge your role. A survey of family caregivers by the National Family Caregivers Association showed that spouse caregivers often refuse to accept that caregiving is a *separate* role to the role of spouse. The survey found that shifting this attitude—accepting that caregiving is a separate role—had a profound impact on their situation.

The job of long-term caregiving is too big for one person— no matter how much love the caregiver has for the care receiver. Ask for and accept help from as many sources as you can find.

Outside Activities

Caregivers must be careful not to give up their own enjoyable activities. Many organizations have respite care programs to provide a break for caregivers, and other family members are often willing to spend time with the care receiver. By asking, it may be possible to have respite care on a regular basis. Keep a list of the people you can ask for help once in a while.

If your friends want to know how they can help ease your burden, ask them to:

- Telephone and be a good listener as you may voice strong feelings

- Offer words of appreciation for your efforts

- Share a meal

- Help you find useful information about community resources

- Stop by for a social visit

- Share the workload

- Help hire a relief caregiver

It helps to remember the saying, "Grant me the serenity to accept the things I cannot change, the courage to change the things I can, and the wisdom to know the difference."

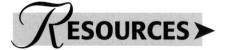

RESOURCES ▸

Caring.com
www.Caring.com
The leading online destination for family caregivers seeking information, support through a community of caregivers and a comprehensive directory of caregiving services.

Taoist Tai Chi Society
www.taoist.org
Membership organization which provides Tai Chi classes nationally and internationally, including a Health Recovery Program for people responding to aging, chronic illness or the consequences of injury. Visit the web site to find a class near you.

Caregiver.com
3350 Griffin Road
Ft. Lauderdale, FL 33312
(800) 829-2734
(954) 893-0550
(954) 893-1779 (fax)
info@caregiver.com
www.caregiver.com or www.caregiver911.com
Publishes Today's Caregiver Magazine. Provides links to many resources, such as government and nonprofit agencies, and information on specific chronic illness. Offers a free Fearless Caregiver Weekly Newsletter focused on caregiver support.

Eldercare Locator
(800) 677-1116
www.eldercarelocator@n4a.org
Provides information about local support resources offering services to the elderly.

Lotsa Helping Hands (calendaring volunteers)
www.lotsahelpinghands.com
Provides a free-of-charge Web service that allows family, friends, neighbors, and colleagues to assist more easily with daily meals, rides, shopping, baby-sitting, and errands that may become a burden during times of medical crisis.

ChooseMyPlate.gov
Provides tips on healthy eating.

National Alliance for Caregiving
4720 Montgomery Lane, 2nd Floor
Bethesda, MD 20814
www.caregiving.org
The Alliance is a non-profit coalition of national organizations focusing on issues of family caregiving.

Caregiver Action Network
2000 M St. NW, Suite 400
Washington, DC 20036
 202-772-5050
www.caregiveraction.org
info@caregiveraction.org
A non-profit organization providing education, peer support, and resources to family caregivers across the country free of charge.

Family Caregiver Alliance, National Center on Caregiving
785 Market Street, Suite 750
San Francisco, CA 94103
(800) 445-8106

If you are providing care to an older or disabled family member or friend, you know that navigating the long-term care system can be difficult. This state-by-state resource is intended to help you locate government, nonprofit, and private programs in your area. It includes services for family caregivers, as well as resources for older or disabled adults living at home or in a residential facility. It also includes information on government health and disability programs, legal resources, disease-specific organizations, and much more. FCA also hosts a number of online support groups.

ARCH National Respite

http://archrespite.org/
Assists and promotes the development of quality respite and crisis care programs in the United States; helps families locate respite and crisis care services in their communities; and serves as a strong voice for respite in all forums.

Well Spouse Association

63 West Main Street, Suite H
Freehold, NJ 07728
(800) 838-0879
(732) 577-8899
(732) 577-8644
info@wellspouse.org
www.wellspouse.org
Publishes *Mainstay*, a quarterly newsletter and provides networking/local support groups.

Check with your local church or health facility to see if they sponsor **caregiver support services.**

Internet - BlogTalk Radio

http://www.blogtalkradio.com/
There's nearly 92 pages of caregiver programs to pick from.

If you don't have home access to the Internet, ask your local library or senior center to help you locate any Web site.

Activities of Daily Living

Activities of Daily Living

Personal Hygiene

As a caregiver, you may find that some of your time each day will be devoted to assisting the person in your care with personal hygiene. This includes bathing, shampooing, oral or mouth care, shaving, and foot care.

The Bed Bath

Bed baths are needed by people who are confined to bed. Baths clean, stimulate, and increase blood flow (circulation) in the skin. However, they can also dry the skin and in some instances cause chapping. Thus, you must decide how often a bed bath is needed. Your decision must be based on the situation of the person in your care. For example, if urinary incontinence (leakage), bowel problems, and heavy perspiration are present, a daily bath may be in order. If not, bathing two to three times a week might be enough. At bath time, inspect the whole body for pressure sores, swelling, rashes, moles, and other unusual conditions. If baths are given often and the skin is dry, use soap and water one time and lotion and water the next. Cornstarch and powder can cause skin problems in some people. Ask the nurse on your health care team for advice.

Skin protectant wipes are used to clean, moisturize, and protect the skin. They are hypoallergenic and easy to use. To prevent skin dryness, use only where the skin needs cleaning.

SKIN CARE
It is easier to prevent chapping than to heal it, so apply lotion often.

To avoid spreading germs, always wash your own hands before and after giving a bath. At each step, tell the person what you are about to do and ask for his help if he is able.

1. Make sure the room is a comfortable temperature and not too warm.

2. Gather supplies—disposable gloves, mild soap, washcloth, washbasin, lotion, comb, electric razor, shampoo—and clean clothes.

3. Use good body mechanics (position)—keep your feet separated, stand firmly, bend your knees, and keep your back in a neutral position. (See p. 336)

4. Offer the bedpan or urinal.

5. If you have a hospital bed, raise the bed to its highest level and bring the head of the bed to an upright position.

6. Help with oral hygiene—brushing the teeth or cleansing the mouth. (See p. 205)

7. Test the temperature of the water in the basin with your hand.

8. Remove the person's clothes, the blanket, and the top sheet. Cover the person with a towel or light blanket. Keep all of the body covered during the bed bath, uncovering only one area at a time while washing it.

9. Now, have the person lie almost flat.

10. Use one washcloth for soap, one for rinsing, and a dry towel. Have the washcloth very damp, but not dripping.

11. Very gently wash the face first; pat dry.

NOTE Always start washing at the cleanest part and work toward the dirtiest part.

12. Wash the front of the neck; pat dry.

13. Wash the chest and, for females, under the breasts; pat dry.

14. Wash the stomach and upper thighs; pat dry.

15. Clean the navel with a little lotion on a cotton swab.

16. Wash upward from wrist to upper arm to increase circulation; pat dry.

17. Wash the hands and between the fingers; check the nails; pat dry.

18. Place a towel under the person's buttocks.

19. Flex (bend) the person's knees.

20. Wash the legs; pat dry.

21. Wash the feet and between the toes and dry well. Use lotion on dry feet. Do not put lotion between toes. This area must be kept dry and clean to prevent fungal infection.

22. Wash the pubic area. If possible, have the person wash his or her own genitals; if not, do it yourself. (Use PeriWash to prevent a buildup of germs.)

23. If a male is not circumcised, draw back the foreskin, rinse, dry, and bring the foreskin down over the head of the penis again. For the female, wash the genitals thoroughly by spreading the external folds. (This must be done at least daily.)

24. Pat the genitals dry.

25. Watch for unusual tenderness, swelling, or hardness in the testicles.

26. Change the bath water.

27. Roll the person away from you.

28. Tuck a towel under the person.

29. Wash the back from the neck to the buttocks.

30. Rinse; dry well.

31. Give a back rub with lotion to improve circulation.

32. Dress the person.

33. Change the bed linens.

34. Trim the toenails and fingernails if they are long.

> **NOTE** A buildup of ear wax may obstruct hearing. Have the ears checked and cleaned by a nurse or doctor twice a year. If the doctor approves, apply a little lotion to the outside of the ears to prevent drying and itching.

The Basin Bath

If the person in your care can sit in a chair or wheelchair, you can give a sponge bath at the sink.

1. Make sure the room is warm.

2. Gather supplies—disposable gloves, mild soap, washcloth, washbasin, lotion, comb, electric razor, shampoo—and clean clothes.

3. Use good body mechanics (position)—keep your feet separated, stand firmly, bend your knees, and keep your back in neutral. (See p. 336)

4. Offer the urinal.

5. Wash the face first.

6. Wash the rest of the upper body.

7. If the person can stand, wash the genitals. If the person is too weak to stand, wash the lower part of the body in the bed.

The Tub Bath

If the person in your care has good mobility and is strong enough to get in and out of the tub, he or she may enjoy a tub bath. Be sure there are grab bars, a bath bench, and a rubber mat so the person doesn't slide. (It may be easier to sit at bench level rather than at the bottom of the tub.) Use the following steps:

1. Make sure the room is a comfortable temperature.

2. Gather supplies—disposable gloves for the caregiver, mild soap, washcloth, lotion, comb, electric razor, shampoo—and clean clothes.

3. Check the water temperature before the person gets in.

4. Guide the person into the tub. Have the person use the grab bars. (Don't let the person grab you and pull you down.)

5. Help the person wash.

6. Empty the tub and then help the person get out.

7. Guide the person to use the grab bars while getting out. OR, you can have the person stand up and then sit on the bath bench. Swing first one leg, then the other leg over the edge of the tub. Help him stand.

8. Put a towel on a chair or the toilet lid and have the person sit there to dry off.

9. Apply lotion to any skin that appears dry.

10. Help the person dress.

> *Tip*
>
> **BATHING IN THE TUB**
> If a bath bench is not used, many people feel more secure if they turn on to their side and then get on their knees before rising from the tub. This is a very helpful way to get out of the tub if the person is unsteady and a bath bench is not available.

The Shower

Before starting, be sure the shower floor is not slippery. Also make sure there are grab bars, a bath bench, and a rubber mat so the person doesn't slide. A removable shower head is also useful.

1. Make sure the room is a comfortable temperature.

2. Explain to the person what you are going to do.

3. Provide a shower stool in case he or she needs to sit.

4. Gather supplies—mild soap, washcloth, washbasin, comb, razor, shampoo—and clean clothes.

5. Turn on the cold water and then the hot to prevent burns. Test and adjust the water temperature before the person gets in. Use gentle water pressure.

6. First, spray and clean the less sensitive parts of the body such as the feet.

7. For safety, ask the person to hold the grab bar or to sit on the shower stool.

8. Move the water hose around the person rather than asking the person to move.

9. Assist in washing as needed.

10. Guide the person out of the shower and wrap with a towel. Turn the water off.

11. Apply lotion to skin that appears dry.

12. If necessary, have the person sit on a stool or on the toilet lid to dry off.

13. Assist in drying and dressing.

 NOTE Remove from the bathing area all electrical equipment that could get wet.

Nail Care

When providing nail care, you can watch for signs of irritation or infection. This is especially important in a person with diabetes, for whom a small infection can develop into something more serious. Fingernails and toenails can thicken with age, which will make them more difficult to trim.

1. Assemble supplies—soap, basin with water, towel, nailbrush, scissors, nail clippers, file, and lotion.

2. Wash your hands.

3. Wash the hands of the person in your care with soap and water and soak the hands in a basin of warm water for 5 minutes.

4. Gently scrub the nails with the brush to remove trapped dirt.

5. Dry the nails and gently push back the skin around the nails (the cuticle) with the towel.

6. To prevent ingrown nails, cut nails straight across.

7. File gently to smooth the edges.

8. Gently massage the person's hands and feet with lotion.

NOTE If other members of the household are using the same grooming supplies, clean the shared items, such as nail clippers, with alcohol.

Shampooing the Hair

Keeping the hair and scalp clean improves blood flow to the scalp and keeps the hair healthy. Shampooing can be done anytime the person in your care is not overly tired. Before a bath may be the most convenient time. Adopt a system that is easiest for you and the person in your care.

Tip **SHAMPOOING**
To make washing easier, dilute the shampoo in a bottle before pouring it on the hair.

Wet Shampoo

1. Assemble supplies—disposable gloves, comb and brush, shampoo/conditioner, several pitchers of warm water, large basin, washcloth, towels.

2. Have the person sit on a chair or commode.

3. Drape a large towel over the person's shoulders.

4. Gently comb out any knots.

5. Protect the person's ears with cotton.

6. Ask the person to cover his or her eyes with a washcloth and to lean over the sink.

7. Moisten the hair with a wet washcloth or with water poured from a pitcher.

8. Massage a small amount of diluted shampoo into the hair.

9. Remove the shampoo with clean water or a washcloth until the rinse water or cloth runs clear.

10. Use a leave-in conditioner if desired.

11. Towel the hair dry.

12. Remove the cotton from the ears.

13. Comb the hair gently.

14. If desired, use a hair dryer on the cool setting to dry hair, being very careful not to burn the scalp.

OR

1. Cut a round slit at the raised edge of a heavy rubber dish-draining mat so that the end can tuck under the person's neck and the water can drain down into the sink.

2. Seat the person at the kitchen sink with her back to the mat.

3. place a towel on the person's shoulders and place the rubber dish-draining mat with the round cut against the neck and the smooth edge draining into the sink (beauty salon style).

4. Follow the procedure above, using the sink hose or a pitcher to wash and rinse the hair.

Dry Shampoo

1. Assemble supplies—disposable gloves for the caregiver, comb and brush, waterless shampoo, and towels.

2. Lather the head until all foam disappears.

3. Towel the hair dry and gently comb it.

Wet Shampoo in Bed

1. Assemble supplies—disposable gloves, comb and brush, shampoo/conditioner, several pitchers of warm water, a large basin, plastic sheet, washcloth, towels, and hair dryer.

2. If possible, raise the bed.

3. Help the person lie flat.

4. Protect the bedding with plastic under the head and shoulders.

5. Roll the edges of the plastic inward so the water will run down into a basin placed on a chair next to the head of the bed.

6. Drape a towel over the person's shoulders.

7. Protect the person's ears with cotton.

8. Cover the person's eyes with a washcloth.

9. Moisten the hair with a wet washcloth.

10. Massage a small amount of diluted shampoo into the hair.

11. Remove the shampoo with a wet washcloth until the water runs clear when the cloth is wrung out.

12. Use leave-in conditioner if desired.

13. Towel the hair dry.

14. Remove the cotton from the ears.

15. Comb the hair gently.

16. Use a hair dryer on the cool setting to dry hair, being very careful not to burn the scalp.

Shaving

Shaving can be done by the person in your care, or you can shave his whiskers with a safety razor or an electric razor. If he wears dentures, make sure they are in his mouth.

1. Assemble supplies—disposable gloves, safety razor, shaving cream, washcloth, towel, lotion.

2. Wash your hands.

3. Adjust the light so that you can clearly see his face but it is not shining in his eyes.

4. Spread a towel under his chin.

5. Soften the beard by wetting the face with a warm, damp washcloth.

6. Apply shaving cream to his face, carefully avoiding the eyes.

7. Hold the skin tight with one hand and using short firm strokes shave in the direction the hair grows.

8. Be careful of sensitive areas.

9. Rinse his skin with a wet washcloth.

10. Pat his face dry with the towel.

11. Apply lotion if the skin appears dry.

 NOTE Never use an electric razor if the person is receiving oxygen because of the risk of causing a fire if the electric razor sparks.

Oral Care

Oral care includes cleaning the mouth and gums and the teeth or dentures. Always be patient and explain what you are about to do. (The person who refuses to brush his teeth can swish and spit out a fluoridated mouthwash rinse.)

1. Gather supplies—disposable gloves, a soft toothbrush or electrical tooth care system, toothpaste or baking soda, warm water in a glass, dental floss, and a bowl.

2. Bring the person to an upright position.

3. If possible, allow the person to clean his or her own teeth. This should be done twice daily and after meals.

4. Be sure the person can spit out water before allowing a sip. Use a water glass for rinsing.

5. If necessary, ask the person to open his or her mouth. Gently brush the front and back teeth up and down.

6. Rinse well by having the person sip water and spit into a bowl.

7. Gently use floss between teeth by standing behind or beside the care receiver.

8. If you have difficulty performing oral care with the person in your care, ask the dentist for pointers.

Oral Care for Someone Who Is Terminally Ill

If your doctor or nurse approves, use hydrogen peroxide diluted with mouthwash or a glycerin/water solution for mouth rinsing. Plain water is best for those who are very sensitive. Your pharmacist can give advice on a gentle mouthwash.

1. Gather supplies—disposable gloves, Toothettes® (foam mouth-swabs), mouthwash, warm water in a glass, and a bowl.

2. Cleanse the mouth (roof, tongue, lips, and cheeks) with the disposable toothbrush.

3. Swab the mouth with a Toothette® dipped in water and repeat until the foam is gone.

4. If the lips are dry, apply a light coat of Vaseline or lip balm.

Denture Cleaning

1. Remove the dentures from the mouth.

2. Run them under water and soak them in cleaner in a denture cup.

3. Rinse the person's mouth with water or mouthwash.

4. Stimulate (massage) the gums with a very soft tooth-brush.

5. Return the dentures to the person's mouth.

 Even a person with dentures should have the soft tissues of the mouth checked regularly by a dentist.

Foot Care

For the comfort and good health of the person in your care:

- Provide properly fitting low-heeled shoes that close with Velcro® or elastic and have nonslip soles. Avoid shoes with heavy soles, running shoes with rubber tips over the toes, and shoes with thick cushioning.

- Provide cotton socks rather than acrylic.

- Trim the person's nails only after a bath, when they have softened.

- Use a disposable sponge-tipped toothbrush to clean or dry between the toes.

- Check feet daily for bumps, cuts, and red spots.

Call the doctor or other health care provider if a sore develops on the foot. The person who is diabetic must have special foot care to prevent infections. Serious infections may result in grave complications or the amputation of a foot.

> **NOTE** Foot pain can cause a person to lean back on the heels. This increases the chance of a fall, so keep toenails trimmed and feet healthy.

Common Leg and Foot Problems and Solutions

Problem	Solution
Foot strain	Visit a podiatrist.
Calluses	Rub lanolin or lotion on the area; do not cut hard skin.
Cramps	Relieve by movement and massage.
Hammer toes and bunions	Wedge a pad between the big toe and the second toe to straighten them; cut holes in the shoe to relieve rubbing.
Leg ulcers (openings in the skin)	Follow the doctor's instructions. Exercise to keep the foot and ankle mobile.
Swollen legs	Follow the doctor's instructions for treatment of the underlying cause.
Varicose veins	Elevate the legs twice a day for 30 minutes. Before lowering the legs, apply an elastic bandage or stocking.

Dressing

Dressing a person with disabilities can be made easier by following a routine. Before you begin, lay the clothes out in the order in which they will be put on.

- Dress the person while he or she is sitting.

- Use adaptive equipment, like a button hook and shoehorn. (See **Equipment and Supplies**, p. 147)

- Use loose clothes that are easy to put on and have elastic waistbands, Velcro® fasteners, and front openings.

- Use bras that open and close in front.

- Use tube socks.

- Dress the weaker side first.

- For a person who is confined to bed, use a gown that closes in the back. This will make it easier when using a bedpan or urinal.

> **NOTE** For a person who is confined to bed, be sure to smooth out all wrinkles in the clothes and bedding to prevent pressure sores.

Bed Making

Making a bed with someone in it will be easier if you follow these steps:

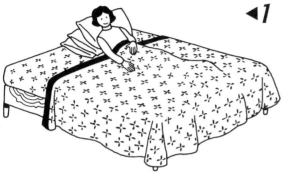

◄**1**
- The bed has two parts—the side the person is lying on and the side you are making.

- If you have a hospital bed, raise the height of the bed.

- Lower the head and foot of the bed so that it is flat.

Draw sheet

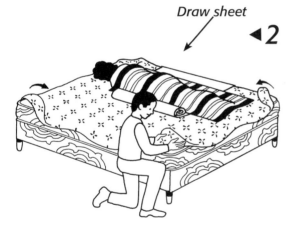

◄**2**
- Loosen the sheets on all sides.

- Remove the blankets and pillow, leaving only the bottom and top sheets.

- Cover the person with a bath blanket (a flannel sheet or large towel) for modesty and warmth.

- Pull the top sheet out from under the bath blanket.

- Raise the bed rail on the side across from you (the opposite side) so the person cannot fall out of bed. If you don't have a hospital bed, be sure the bed is pushed against the wall.

- Roll the person over to the opposite side of the bed.

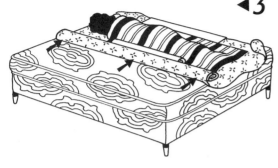

◀3 • Roll all the old bottom sheeting toward the person.

Clean sheet

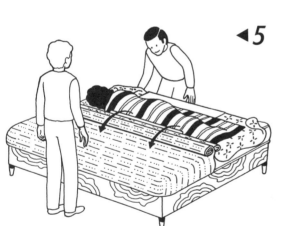

◀4 • Fold the clean sheet, along with other mattress covers, lengthwise.

• Place it on the bed with the middle fold running along the center of the mattress, right beside the person's body.

◀5 • Unfold the clean sheet and bring enough of it toward you to cover half of the bed.

• Gently lift the mattress and tuck the sheet in.

• Tuck the free edge of the draw sheet under the mattress on your side of the bed.

• Ask the person to roll over the linens in the middle of bed to the clean side.

OR

- Bend as close to the person's body as possible. Place your hand and arm under the person's shoulders and move the person and the bath blanket over the linens in the center of the bed.

- If it is a hospital bed, raise the bed rail on your side and lock it into place.

- Go to the other side and remove all soiled linen. Tuck in all the linen and pull tight on the sheets to remove all wrinkles so they don't rub and irritate the person's skin.

- Change the pillowcase.

- Spread the top sheet over the person and bath blanket.

- Ask the person to hold the sheet while you pull the bath blanket away.

- Tuck the sheet under the mattress at the foot of the bed.

◀**6**

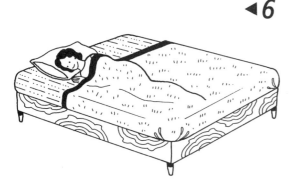

- Spread a blanket over the top. (The blanket should be up far enough to cover the person's shoulders.)

- Fold the sheet down over the blanket.

- Adjust the person in bed so he or she is comfortable.

Toileting

Always wear disposable gloves when helping with toileting. This prevents the spread of disease. Wash your hands before and after providing care.

Toileting in Bed

When a person is mobile, toileting in bed should not be encouraged.

Toileting in Bed for a Female or for Bowel Movements

1 • Wash your hands and put gloves on.

• Warm the bedpan with warm water. Empty the water into the toilet.

• Powder the bedpan with talcum powder to keep the skin from sticking to it.

• Place a tissue or water in the pan to make cleaning easier. Or use a light spray of vegetable oil in the bedpan, which will make it easier to empty the contents.

• Raise the person's gown.

◄*2* • Ask the person to raise her hips.

◀**3** • If the person cannot raise her hips, turn her on her side and roll the hips back onto the bedpan.

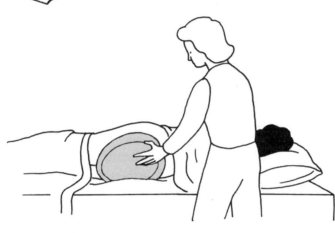

▲**4**

• If the person cannot do so, clean the anal area with bathroom tissue. Then use a wet tissue to clean the area.

• After the woman has urinated, pour a cup of warm water over her genitals and pat the area dry with a towel.

• Remove and empty the bedpan.

• Remove your gloves and wash your hands.

• Wash the person's hands and rewash your hands.

Using a Urinal

1. If the person can't do so himself, put gloves on and place the penis into the urinal as far as possible and hold it in.

2. When the person signals he is finished, remove and empty the urinal.

3. Remove your gloves and wash your hands.

4. Wash his hands, then rewash your hands.

Using a Commode

A portable commode is helpful for a person with limited mobility. The portable commode (with the pail removed) can be used over the toilet seat and as a shower seat.

Using a Portable Commode

1. Gather the portable commode, toilet tissue, a basin, a cup of water, a washcloth or paper towel, soap, and a towel.

2. Wash your hands and put on gloves

3. Help the person onto the commode.

4. Offer toilet tissue when the person is finished.

5. Pour a cup of warm water on female genitalia.

6. Pat the area dry with a paper towel.

7. Remove the pail from under the seat, empty it, rinse it with clear water, and empty the water into the toilet.

8. Remove your gloves and wash your hands.

9. Offer a washcloth so the person can wash his or her hands.

> ## TOILET SAFETY
> *Tip*
>
> Use Velcro® with tape on the back and attach it to the back of the toilet or commode seat to keep the lid from falling.

Using the Bathroom Toilet

If the mobile person is missing the toilet, get a toilet seat in a color that is different from the floor color. This may help him see the toilet better. If he is failing to cleanse the anal area or failing to wash his hands, use tact to encourage him to do so. This will help prevent the spread of infections.

Catheters

A urinary catheter is a device made from rubber or plastic that drains urine from the body. It is inserted by a nurse through the urethra (a tube that connects the bladder to the outside of the body) into the bladder (an organ that collects urine).

A Foley catheter stays in the bladder and drains into a bag that is attached to a person's leg, the bed, or a chair. When caring for someone with this kind of catheter (called an indwelling catheter), watch for these things:

1. Be sure the tube stays straight and drains properly. Check for kinks in the tubing.

2. Be sure the level of urine in the bag increases.

3. Be sure the drainage bag is always lower than the bladder.

4. Use tape or straps when securing a catheter to someone's inner thigh.

5. In males, an erection is a common effect when a catheter is inserted.

6. Tell the doctor if blood or sediment (matter that settles to the bottom) appears in the tubing or bag.

 A Foley catheter greatly increases the risk of infection. It is a last resort to manage incontinence (leaking of urine or inability to control bowel movements).

Care of the Person Who Has a Catheter

1. Wash your hands.

2. Put on disposable gloves.

3. Position the person on his or her back.

4. Take care not to pull on the catheter.

5. While holding the catheter, wash the area around it with a washcloth.

6. To avoid infection, wipe toward the anus, not back and forth.

7. Remove gloves and wash your hands

 To prevent foul odors due to the growth of bacteria in the urine drainage bag, put a few drops of hydrogen peroxide in the bag when it is emptied.

Changing a Catheter from Straight Drainage to Leg Bag

1. Gather supplies—disposable gloves, a bed protector, alcohol wipes, and a leg bag with straps.

2. Uncover the end of the catheter and draining tubing; put a towel or other bed protector under this area.

3. Put on gloves.

4. Disconnect the drainage tubing from the catheter.

5. Wipe the attachment tube of the leg bag with an alcohol swab and insert it into the catheter.

6. Place the cap attached to the urinary drainage bag over the end of the tubing to keep it clean and prevent urine from leaking out.

7. Secure the tubing to the person's leg.

8. Remove gloves and wash hands.

Condom Catheter

The doctor may prescribe a condom catheter for a male if infections from the indwelling catheter become a chronic problem. The catheter fits over the penis like a condom. Leakage is often a problem with this type of aid. **It is extremely important that a condom catheter not be secured too tightly, which can result in serious injury**. Other products for male incontinence are available that are less constricting, such as Bio Derm's Liberty Pouch, which uses "skin friendly" adhesive.

Incontinence

Incontinence is the leakage of urine or a bowel movement over which the person has no control. In addition to bladder management medications, treatments can include bladder training, exercises to strengthen the pelvic floor (Kegel exercises), biofeedback, surgery, electrical muscle stimulator, urinary catheter, prosthetic devices, or external collection devices. Talk to the doctor about the options or treatments for the person in your care.

To Manage Incontinence

- Avoid alcohol, coffee, spicy foods, and citrus foods. These can irritate the bladder and can increase the need to urinate.

- Give fluids at regular intervals to dilute the urine. This decreases the irritation of the bladder.

- Be sure the person in your care voids (goes to the bathroom) regularly, ideally every 2 to 3 hours. Use an alarm clock to keep track of the time.

- Provide clothing that can be easily removed.

- Keep a bedpan or a portable commode near the person.

- Provide absorbent products (adult diapers) to be worn under clothes.

- Stroke or tap the lower abdomen to cause voiding.

- Keep the skin dry and clean. Urine on the skin can cause pressure sores and infection.

- Your patience and understanding will help the person have confidence and self-respect.

NOTE A precise diagnosis for incontinence must be made in order to come up with an effective treatment plan. If the primary care doctor cannot solve the problem, consult an experienced urologist.

Urinary Tract Infection

Urinary tract infection may be present if the person has any of the following signs or symptoms:

- Blood in the urine

- A burning feeling when voiding

- Cloudy urine with sediment (matter that settles to the bottom)

- Pain in the lower abdomen or lower back

- Fever and chills

- Foul-smelling urine

- A frequent, strong urge to void or frequent voiding

Get in touch with the doctor if there is any sign of a urinary tract infection.

Optimal Bowel Function

Maintaining good bowel function can be a challenge, especially in individuals who are unable to get out of bed and get little exercise. For optimal bowel function—

- Set a time for bowel movements every day or every other day. The best time is 20–30 minutes after breakfast.

- Serve fruits, vegetables, and bran.

- Be sure the person in your care drinks 2 quarts (8 glasses) of water daily (or an amount directed by the doctor).

- Provide a chance for daily exercise.

- Use a stool softener or bulk agent if the stools are too hard. When using a bulk laxative, be sure that 6 to 8 glasses of water are taken per day. This will lessen the chance of severe constipation.

- Use glycerin suppositories as needed to help lubricate the bowels for ease of movement.

- Massage the abdomen in a clockwise direction. This can stimulate a bowel movement.

- Avoid laxatives and enemas unless specifically ordered by the doctor or nurse.

Diarrhea

Diarrhea (loose, watery stools) occurs when the intestines push stool along before the water in them can be reabsorbed (taken up) by the body. This condition can be caused by viral stomach flu, antibiotics, or other medications, or stress anxiety.

Diarrhea in people who are immobile is often caused by impaction. This is a blockage formed by hardened stool, with liquid stool passing around it. This must always be taken into consideration, because the usual treatments for diarrhea would be extremely dangerous if the diarrhea is being caused by impaction.

To counteract diarrhea, consider two types of antidiarrheals:

- Those that thicken the stool

- Those that slow intestinal spasms

Ask the pharmacist for advice.

Precautions:

- Do not use for the first 6 hours after diarrhea begins.

- Do not use if fever is present.

- Stop taking as soon as stool thickens.

- Encourage fluid to prevent dehydration.

Hemorrhoids

Hemorrhoids are swollen inflamed veins around the anus. They cause tenderness, pain, and bleeding. To treat hemorrhoids, you should do the following:

- Be sure to keep anal area clean with premoistened tissues.

- Apply zinc oxide or petroleum jelly to the area.

- Relieve itching by using cold compresses on the anus for 10 minutes several times a day.

- Ask the doctor about suppositories.

Call the Doctor

- If blood from the hemorrhoids is dark red or brown and heavy

- If bleeding continues for more than one week

- If bleeding seems to occur for no reason

Control of Infection in the Home

Common health practices, such as frequent hand-washing, are necessary to avoid the risk of bacterial, viral, and fungal infections.

NOTE To minimize the chance of infection
- Always start with the cleanest area and work toward the dirtiest area.
- Always wash your hands before and after contact with the person in your care and with other people.
- Always wear disposable gloves when giving personal care.
- Always wash hands well when returning from a trip outside the house.
- Always wash your hands after using the toilet.
- Keep a travel-size hand sanitizer with you.

Cleaning Techniques

The following techniques will help cut the chance of infection in the home.

Caregiver Hand-Washing

- Hand-washing is the single most effective way to prevent the spread of infection or germs.

- Use bottle-dispensed hand soap.

- If the person in your care has an infection, use antimicrobial soap.

- Rub your hands for at least 30 seconds to produce lots of lather. Do this away from running water so that the lather is not washed away.

- Use a nailbrush on your nails; keep nails trimmed.

- Wash front and back of hands, between fingers, and at least 2 inches up your wrists.

- Repeat the process.

- Dry your hands on a clean towel or a paper towel.

Precautions for Anyone Who Propels His Own Wheelchair

- Wear leather gloves.

- Wash your hands frequently.

- For frequent in-between washings, use prepackaged cleansing towelettes.

Handling Soiled Laundry

- Do not carry soiled linen close to your body.

- Never shake dirty items or put soiled linens on the floor. They can contaminate (infect) the floor, and germs will be spread throughout the house on the soles of shoes.

- Store infected soiled linen in a leak-proof plastic bag and tie it closed.

- Bag soiled laundry in the same place it is used.

- Wash soiled linen separately from other clothes.

- Fill the machine with hot water, add bleach (no more than 1/4 cup) and detergent. Rinse twice and then dry.

- Clean the washer by running it through a cycle with 1 cup of bleach or other disinfectant to kill germs.

- Use rubber gloves when handling soiled laundry.

- Wash your hands.

 If urine is highly concentrated due to a bladder infection or dehydration, do not use bleach. The combination of ammonia in the urine and bleach can cause toxic fumes.

Sterilization

If you are sharing equipment with other members of the family, sterilizing will cut down on infection. If you are not sharing equipment, wiping it with a cotton ball soaked in alcohol is adequate. Sterilization is a process that destroys bacteria.

Wet Heat Sterilization

1. Fill a large pot with water.

2. If sterilizing glass items, put a cloth in the bottom of the pot to prevent breakage.

3. Put items to be sterilized in the pot. These might include syringes, nail trimmers, and scissors.

4. Cover the pot and bring the water to a boil.

5. Boil, covered, for 20 minutes.

6. Leave the items in the pot until ready to use.

Steam Sterilization

Steam sterilization is the most common and preferred method for sterilization of all items that penetrate the skin and mucosa. Steam sterilization is dependable, non-toxic, and inexpensive. It's quick and can be used to sterilize fabrics as well. Online, you can find inexpensive handheld steam cleaners that reach a temperature of over 212°F. This temperature (the boiling point of water) kills germs, bacteria, and dust mites.

NOTE Cloth can be sterilized by holding a hot iron on it for a few seconds. Never use the microwave oven to disinfect (kill germs) any nonfood items. They can catch fire or explode.

Disposal of Body Fluids

- Wear disposable gloves (recommended for handling all body fluids).

- Flush liquid and solid waste down the toilet.

- Place used dressings and disposable (throwaway) pads in a sturdy plastic bag, tie securely, and place in a sealed container for collection.

Prevention of Odors Caused by Bacteria

Bacteria need moisture, warmth, oxygen, darkness, and nourishment to grow. Some strong odors may be eliminated by

- Sprinkling baking soda on discarded wound dressing

- Leaving an open can of finely ground coffee under the bed

- Pouring a few drops of mouthwash in commodes and bedpans

- Placing cotton balls soaked in mouthwash in the room

- Spraying a fine mist of white distilled vinegar mixed with a few drops of eucalyptus or peppermint essential oil around the room

- Soaking cotton balls with vanilla extract and placing them in any containers that hold on to strong odors

- Using electrical and mechanical devices, such as plug-in air fresheners and fans, for removing odor. (Be aware that commercial air fresheners contain chemical compounds that could aggravate breathing problems in people with COPD or asthma.)

- Making a pomander. Stud an orange with whole cloves and cure it in the oven on low heat for about an hour (or place it in a paper bag somewhere cool and dry for about 6 weeks).

- Opening the windows. Every house benefits from a good airing out. On a day with good air quality and a slight breeze, open windows for a few hours on all sides of the house to create a cross breeze that gets air moving.

- Simmering spices such as whole cinnamon, cloves, and nutmeg on the stovetop or in a simmering pot.

- Placing a box of baking soda to absorb odors in especially smelly spots.

- Using white vinegar to clean and remove odors from surfaces.

- Buying natural organic room sprays or potpourri

Skin Care and Prevention of Pressure Sores

Pressure sores (also called decubiti, or bedsores) are blisters or breaks in the skin. They are caused when the body's weight presses blood out of a certain area. The best treatment of pressure sores is prevention. How much time they take to heal depends on how advanced they are.

Facts

- The most common areas for sores are the bony areas— tailbone, hips, heels, and elbows.

- Sores can appear when the skin keeps rubbing on a sheet.

- The skin breakdown starts from the inside, works up to the surface, and can happen in just 15 minutes.

- Damage can range from a change in color in unbroken skin to deep wounds down to the muscle or bone.

- For people with light skin in the first stage of a bedsore, the skin color may change to dark purple or red that does not turn pale under fingertip pressure. For people with dark skin, this area may become darker than normal.

- The affected area may feel warmer than the skin around it.

- Pressure sores that are not treated can lead to hospitalization and can require skin grafts.

Prevention

- Check the skin daily. (Bath time is the ideal time to do this.)

- Provide a well-balanced diet, with enough vitamin C, zinc, and protein.

- Keep the skin dry and clean (urine left on the skin can cause sores and infection).

- Keep clothing loose.

- If splints or braces are used, make sure they are adjusted properly.

- Massage the body with light pressure, using equal parts surgical spirit and glycerin. (Ask a nurse or a pharmacist for advice.)

- Turn a person who is unable to get out of bed at least every 2 hours. Change the person's positions. Smooth wrinkles out of sheets.

- Lightly tape foam to bony sections of the body using paper tape, which will not hurt the skin when peeled off.

- Use flannel or 100% cotton sheets to absorb moisture.

- Provide an egg-crate or sheepskin mattress pad for added comfort.

- Rent an electrically operated ripple bed. These beds have sections that can be inflated separately and at different times.

- Avoid using a plastic sheet or a Chux if they cause sweating.

- When the person is sitting, encourage changing the body position every 15 minutes.

- Use foam pads on chair seats to cushion the buttocks.

- Change the type of chair the person sits in; try an open-back garden chair occasionally.

- Provide as much exercise as possible.

WOUND PREVENTION

If a person tends to scratch or pick at a spot, have the person wear cotton gloves. (Make sure the hands are clean and dry before putting the gloves on.)

When Turning Someone in Bed to Minimize Sores

1. Explain to the person what you are doing.

2. If possible, raise the bed to its highest position.

3. Lower the head of the bed to a flat position.

4. Loosen the draw sheet at the far side.

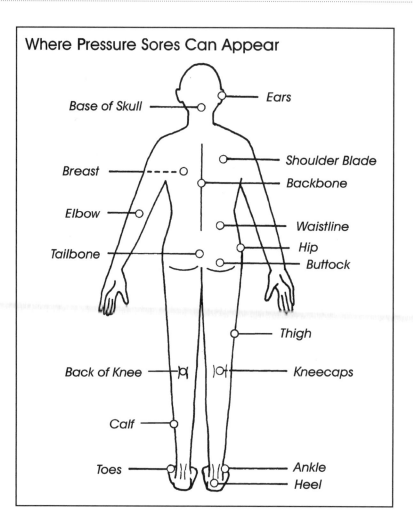

Where Pressure Sores Can Appear

Ears
Base of Skull
Shoulder Blade
Breast
Backbone
Elbow
Waistline
Hip
Tailbone
Buttock
Thigh
Back of Knee
Kneecaps
Calf
Toes
Ankle
Heel

5. Stand in proper position as close to the person as possible.

6. Roll the far side of the draw sheet toward you and up close to the person's side.

7. Prop a pillow against the person's back.

8. Flex the person's knees slightly.

9. Place one pillow between the knees and another between the feet.

10. Check any catheter tubing.

Treatment

If you see pressure sores in your daily checking of the skin, you must alert the nurse or the doctor. General guidelines for treatment of these sores are as follows:

• To reduce the chance of infection, wear disposable gloves at all times when providing care.

• Take pressure off sores by changing the person's position often. Use pillows or a foam pad with at least 1 inch of padding to support the body.

• Do not position the person on his or her bony parts.

• Do not let the person lie on pressure sores.

• In bed, change the person's position at least every 2 hours.

• Follow the doctor's or nurse's treatment plan in applying medication to sores and bandaging the areas to protect them while they heal.

Eating

Mealtimes are important because they provide a welcome break in the day. If it is not too distracting for the person in your care, meals can be eaten with friends or family. It is important that mealtimes be enjoyable so that the person will look forward to eating.

Look for these free or low-cost solutions:

Community meals—local meal programs sponsored by the federal government and open to those who are eligible. Some meal locations do not require an income limit as long as you are a resident of the community. Call the local Area Agency on Aging or Department of Health and Human Resources, your local independent Living Center, or Senior Center

Meals-on-Wheels—hot meals delivered to the home. Call your local county office of Health and Human Services or Aging and Disability Council.

Food stamps—help based on income that can stretch food dollars. Call the Department of Health and Human Resources or the Area Agency on Aging.

For best results at mealtime:

- Allow 30 to 45 minutes for eating.

- Avoid fussy meal presentation.

- Make sure all items are ready to eat and within reach.

- Provide a comfortable table and chair or other eating arrangement.

- Supply easy-to-hold eating utensils. To avoid cuts, throw out all chipped cups and plates.

- Reduce excess noise such as TV and radio.

- If the person's vision is poor, place the same foods in the same spot on the plate every time.

Feeding Someone in Bed

1. Prop the head with pillows.

2. Provide an over-the-bed table.

3. Do not rush feeding, but maintain a steady pace.

4. Cut the food into bite-size portions.

5. Fill cups only halfway.

6. Let the person hold the cup if he or she wants to. (A terry cloth tennis wristband slipped over the cup may make it easier to hold.)

7. Use available eating aids. (📖 See **Equipment and Supplies**, p. 146)

8. Keep a moist hand towel to wipe the person's mouth and hands gently. The chains used to hang eyeglasses around the neck can be used to hold a napkin in place.

> *Tip*
>
> **FEEDING IN BED**
> An adjustable ironing board may be used as an over-the-bed table for activities or eating.

Feeding the Person Who Is Disabled

1. Name the food being offered, if necessary.

2. If the person plays with food, limit the choices being offered. (Playing with food occurs because a person is distracted, confused, or unable to make choices.)

3. Check the temperature of the food often.

4. Be gentle with forks and spoons. (A rubber-tipped baby spoon may be helpful.)

5. Feed at a steady pace, alternating food with drink.

6. Remove a spoon from the person's mouth very slowly. If the person clenches the spoon, let go of it and wait for the jaw to relax.

7. Give simple instructions such as "Open your mouth," "Move your tongue," "Now swallow."

8. If the person spits food out, try feeding later.

9. If the person refuses food, provide a drink and return in 10 minutes with the food tray.

10. Between meals, provide a nourishing snack, such as stewed fruit, tapioca pudding, or finger foods. Supplement drinks can provide needed nourishment between meals, as a snack or supplement to add calories to the senior's diet—not as a meal replacement.

Boosting Food Intake When the Appetite Is Poor

- Offer more food at the time of day when the person is most hungry or less tired.

- To increase the appeal of food for those with decreased taste and smell, provide strong flavors.

- Use milk or cream instead of water in soups and cooked cereal.

- Add saturated fat by using butter, non-trans fat margarines, or olive oil on foods.

- Add nonfat dry-milk powder to foods like yogurt, mashed potatoes, gravy, and sauces.

- Tell the person to eat with his or her fingers if that is the only way to get the person to eat.

- Offer milk or fruit shakes.

- Offer puréed (finely ground) baby foods.

(📖 See *Diet, Nutrition, and Exercise*, p. 283)

> **NOTE** If the person in your care needs to swallow three or four times with each bite of food; coughs before, during, or after swallowing; pockets food in the mouth; or senses something caught or sticking in the back of the throat, he or she may have a condition called *dysphagia*. Difficulty swallowing must be evaluated to determine if it is a symptom of a treatable condition and to help the caregiver learn proper feeding techniques. Seek the advice of the doctor.

Eating Problems and Solutions

Drooling—Use a straw if possible; help close the mouth with your hand. (However, sometimes the use of a straw can cause choking if liquid touches the back of the mouth too quickly.)

Spitting out food—Ask the doctor if the cause is moodiness or disease.

Too much swallowing or chewing—Coach the person to alternate hot and cold bites.

Difficulty chewing—Change the diet to soft foods.

Difficulty swallowing—Put foods through a blender or food mill; avoid thin liquids and instead serve thick liquids, such as milk shakes.

Poor scooping—Use bowls instead of plates.

Difficulty cutting food—Use a small pizza cutter or rolling knife.

Trouble moving food to the back of the mouth—Change the food's thickness and demonstrate how to direct the food to the center of the mouth.

Too dry or too wet mouth—Ask the doctor or the pharmacist if this is a side effect of medications.

Too easily distracted—Pull down the shades and remove the distractions.

 Difficulty in swallowing can cause food or liquids to be taken into the lungs, which can lead to pneumonia. Reduce the chance of food entering the lungs by keeping the person upright for at least 30 minutes after a meal.

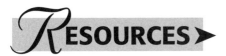

Meeting Life's Challenges
9042 Aspen Grove Lane
Madison, WI 53717
Fax (608) 824-0403
www.makinglifeeasier.com
help@makinglifeeasier.com

Offers numerous tips and strategies for dealing with day-to-day aspects of caregiving, chronic illness, and aging.

National Association for Continence (NAFC)
P.O. Box 1019
Charleston, SC 29402-1019
(800) 252-3337
(843) 377-0900
(843) 377-0905 (fax)
memberservices@nafc.org
www.nafc.org
NAFC is a leading source of education and support to the public about the diagnosis, treatments, and management alternatives for incontinence

Mayo Clinic Web Page on Nutrition
http://www.mayoclinic.com/health/nutrition-and-healthy-eating/MY00431
Although it is true that what is known about nutrition and diet is evolving, there are some nutrition basics you can keep in mind. By knowing these nutrition basics, you'll be better equipped to sort through the latest research and advice.

If you don't have home access to the Internet, ask your local library or senior center to help you locate any Web site.

Therapies

Therapies

The following information is provided for your general knowledge. It IS NOT a substitute for training with professional therapists.

Physical Therapy

Physical therapy is part of the process of relearning how to function after an injury, illness, or period of inactivity. If muscles are not used, they shorten and tighten, making joint motion painful.

What a Physical Therapist Does

A physical therapist treats a person to relieve pain, build up and restore muscle function, and maintain the best possible performance. The therapist does this by using physical means such as active and passive exercise, massage, heat, water, and electricity. Broadly speaking, a physical therapist:

- Sets up the goals of treatment with patient and family
- Shows how to use special equipment
- Instructs in routine daily functions
- Teaches safe ways to move
- Sets up and teaches an exercise program

 NOTE The American Physical Therapy Association, often located in the state capital, can provide a list of licensed therapists.

What a Physical Therapist Determines

Depending on a person's physical condition, a therapist may work on range-of-motion exercises, correct body positions when resting, devices to help the person in your care, and other simple ways to improve daily functions.

A physical therapist checks things that can affect a person's daily activities—

• The person's attitude toward his situation

• How well he can move his muscles and joints (range of motion)

• His ability to see, smell, hear, and feel

• What he can do on his own and what he needs to learn

• His equipment needs, now and in the future

• What can be improved in the home to make moving around safer and more comfortable

• Who can and will help to give support

Range-of-Motion (ROM) Exercises

The purpose of range-of-motion exercises is to relieve pain, maintain normal body alignment (positions), help prevent skin swelling and breakdown, and promote bone formation. A ROM exercise program should be started before deformities develop. Here are some things to do when you are asked to help with exercises at home:

• Communicate what you are doing.

• Use the flats of both hands, not the fingertips, to hold a body part.

• Take each movement only as far as the joint will go into a comfortable stretch. (Mild discomfort is okay, but it should go away quickly.)

Joints Used in ROM

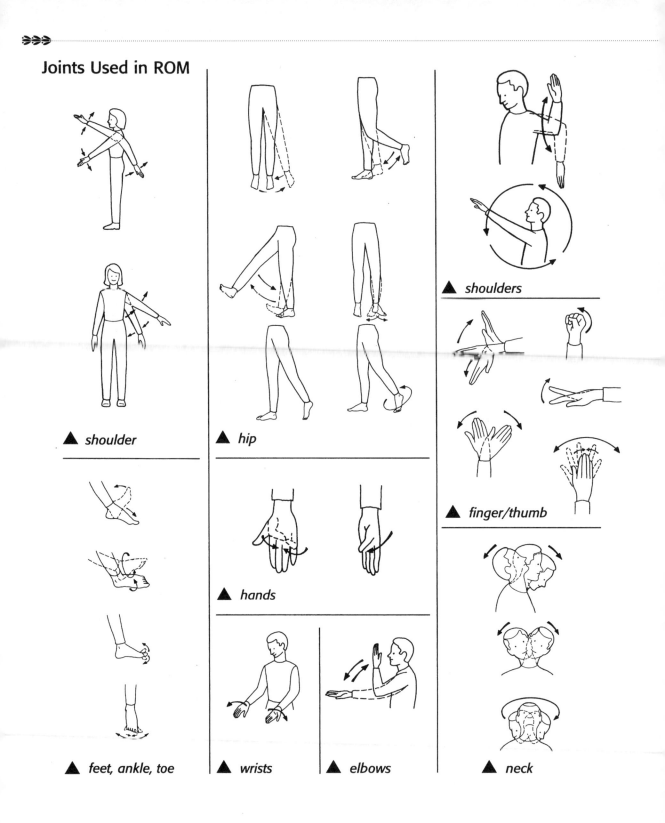

▲ shoulder

▲ hip

▲ shoulders

▲ finger/thumb

▲ hands

▲ feet, ankle, toe

▲ wrists

▲ elbows

▲ neck

- Do each exercise 3 to 5 times.

- Use slow steady movements to help relax muscles and increase joint range.

- If joints are swollen and painful, exercise very gently.

Proper Positions to Use When Resting:

- Flat on the back or no more than 30 degrees raised

- Prone (lying flat) on the stomach (for up to 20 to 30 minutes only, not for sleeping)

- One-quarter left or right turn onto the back

- Three-quarters right or left turn on to the stomach

- Aided by special positioning devices (for example, splints for leg, foot, hand, or back support)

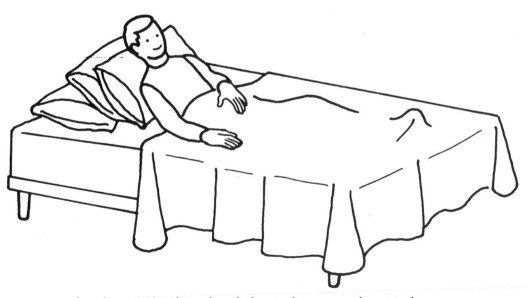

▲ *When resting keep head elevated no more than 30 degrees.*

Positioning Devices for Stroke Patients

Arm Trough—attaches to the arm of a wheelchair; provides support and positioning of the arm

Finger Spreader—keeps the hand in a relaxed position with the fingers spread

Lap Board—lies across both arms of a wheelchair; provides support and positioning

Resting Hand Splint—slowly relaxes muscles; keeps the hand in an open position with the thumb away from the palm

Shoulder Girdle Sling—holds the shoulder joint in a normal position

Sling—supports a flaccid arm (rarely used now)

Occupational Therapy

Occupational therapy is designed to help people regain and build skills that are important for functioning on their own. The occupational therapist will help the person evaluate levels of function.

The occupational therapist will—

- Test a person's strength, range of motion, endurance (the ability to continue an activity or effort), and dexterity (skill in using hands) to do everyday tasks that were done easily before an illness or injury happened

- Design a program of activities and solutions that ensure the greatest possible independence

- Provide training to relearn everyday activities of daily living like eating, grooming, dressing, toileting, bathing, and leisure activities

- Decide whether special equipment is needed, such as wheelchairs, feeding devices, transfer equipment, hand and skin devices

Speech Therapy

Speech therapy is the treatment of disorders that involve speaking, hearing, writing, reading, and other communication required for the activities of daily living. Speech therapists also teach people to swallow foods and liquids safely.

A speech therapist or speech pathologist works to—

- Strengthen weakened oral muscles through exercises

- Teach methods of basic communication

- Teach a patient and family how to manage a communication or swallowing disorder

Specialized Therapies

Many types of therapy exist to help with special needs, both in the hospital and at home. They include:

Antibiotic Therapy—antibiotics infused into a vein to treat lingering infections

Chemotherapy—anti-cancer medication given through a lightweight infusion pump

Dialysis—machines to clean the blood in the case of kidney failure

Enteral Nutrition Therapy—liquid nutrition pumped through a thin feeding tube from the nose into the stomach or surgically placed into the small intestine by way of the abdomen

Enterostomal Therapy—training in the care of hard-to-heal sores, wounds, and ostomy (an artificial opening in the abdomen for the removal of urine and stool)

Infusion Therapy—fluids for nutrition, antibiotics, or chemotherapy given intravenously

Respiratory Therapy—oxygen systems that help with breathing problems and keep lung function at its highest level

Total Parenteral Nutrition (TPN)—infusion of nutrients through a vein for one who cannot eat

Massage Therapy

Massage therapy is an aid to good health because it relaxes muscles, increases blood flow, and releases stress. You can learn to give a simple massage; however, massage for cancer, HIV or AIDS-afflicted persons should be done only by a professional. Never massage broken skin.

When you give a massage, use only natural oils (olive or almond). Never use mineral oils or petroleum-based products like Vaseline.

Back Massage

- Wash your hands with warm water.

- Use warm massage oil or baby powder.

- Expose the back to the top of the buttocks.

- Apply oil to the entire back from shoulders to buttocks with long firm strokes.

- Use gentle circular motions on each area.

- Dry the back.

Hand Massage

- Wash your hands with warm water.

- Apply warm massage oil or lotion.

- Use short or medium strokes from wrist to fingertips.

- Gently squeeze all sides of the fingers from base to tip. Use this "milking" motion on the entire hand.

- Lay the person's hand on yours and gently draw your top hand toward you several times.

- Do not massage portions of the hand that are swollen or red.

TREATING INFLAMMATION

If the finger joints are inflamed, apply ice for the first 24 hours and provide an anti-inflammatory pain reliever, unless the person's physician has not recommended it.

Acupuncture

Acupuncture is a form of treatment used in traditional Chinese medicine. It is based on the theory that the body contains a flow of energy. Acupuncture involves stimulating certain locations on the skin by inserting thin, disposable, metallic needles into points along the meridians (or pathways) in the body in order to alter the flow of energy. Similar methods include finger pressure, cupping with small heated cups, and electroacupuncture with electrically stimulated needles.

Acupuncture is a safe treatment for most people. It is important to remember that acupuncture must be combined with standard medical treatment.

Horticultural Therapy

Gardening is one of the oldest healing arts. The goal is to improve mental and physical health and the person's spirits.

Advantages of Horticultural Therapy

Horticultural therapy—

- Exercises eyes and body

- Provides leisure activities when the person can no longer do other activities

- Promotes interest and enthusiasm for the future

- Provides something to talk about

- Encourages a person to walk and bend

- Improves confidence

- Provides a feeling of being useful

- Allows time to daydream

- Makes it possible to grow useful house plants or vegetables

- Allows a person to be in the sun and enjoy the soothing sounds of nature

To Make Gardening Easier

Make sure that proper body mechanics (positions) are used. Avoid twisting the body, face in the direction of the work being done, and lift using the strength of the upper body and legs. A weightlifter's belt can provide back support.

- Use proper equipment and tools that are right for the person's height and strength.

- Avoid sunburn, chemicals, and hazardous plants.

- Use raised beds to avoid stooping or bending.

- Use perennials, which do not have to be planted every year.

- Use seed tape or mechanical seeders to reduce the need to hold tiny seeds in the hand.

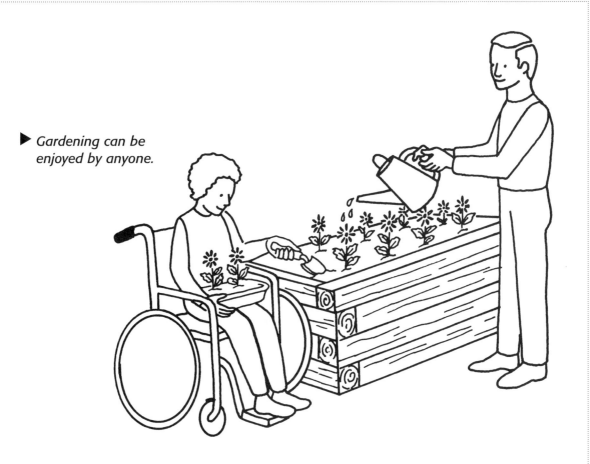

▶ *Gardening can be enjoyed by anyone.*

- Ensure that gardening walkways are 3 feet wide and have nonslip surfaces.

- For those with arthritis, provide gloves that are large enough for foam inserts. The foam eases pain.

- Use tools with cushioned grips.

- Provide foam pads for kneeling or a small stool for sitting.

- To help prevent knee injury, avoid a squatting position. Have the person in your care sit on the ground and move backwards.

- Provide a timer as a reminder to change body position every 20 minutes to avoid repetitive motions.

> **NOTE** If the person in your care is in the garden alone, provide a whistle on a cord worn around the neck or another noise-making device so he or she can call for help.

Aromatherapy

Aromatherapy is a branch of herbal medicine that uses the oils of various plants for medicinal (healing) purposes. These essential oils act to boost energy or calm, aid digestion, and remove toxins (poisons) from the body.

Ways to Use Essential Oils

- With a diffuser—for those with some respiratory conditions

- Through outer application—in baths or with massages (2 or 3 drops with almond or olive oil)

- In floral waters—sprayed on skin that is too sensitive to touch

Common Conditions to Treat with Essential Oils

- For insomnia, a room perfumed with lavender or rose in a diffuser is an effective treatment. (A diffuser is a device that creates a mist.)

- For low energy, use geranium and peppermint.

- For relaxation, try cinnamon and chamomile in a diffuser or rubbed on the wrists and temples.

- For pleasant thoughts, try the aroma of ginger, cloves, and allspice.

- To cleanse the respiratory system (lungs, air passages), use eucalyptus in a diffuser.

Essential oils can be expensive but they last a long time. Buy essential oils from a supplier or a health food store. Starter kits with the most widely used selections are available. **Never drink essential oils or use them directly on the skin.**

 People with medical conditions should consult their health professional before using essential oils.

Pet Therapy

A cat, bird, or dog can bring great joy to people. They provide companionship, relaxation, and a chance to exercise. They also lessen the boredom and fear caused by loneliness.

- Before selecting a dog, check canine-assistant programs in your area. Dogs that were rejected from the program may be ideal for the person in your care.

- Choose a mature dog that is housetrained; do not get a puppy.

- Have a dog or cat neutered or spayed to lessen the chance of roaming.

- Keep up all pet vaccinations.

- Never clean pet cages or feeding dishes in the kitchen sink.

 Be aware that animals carry bacteria and intestinal para- sites. Individuals with weakened immune systems should not change the litter box or pick up outside waste and should wash their hands frequently.

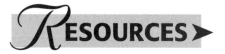

RESOURCES

Acufinder.com
909 North Sepulveda Boulevard, 11th Floor
El Segundo, CA 90245
(760) 630-3600
www.acufinder.com
A referral service that lists state-licensed acupuncturists.

American Academy of Medical Acupuncture
1970 E. Grand Avenue, Suite 330
El Segundo, CA 90245
(310) 364-0193
www.medicalacupuncture.org

American Horticultural Therapy Association
610 Freedom Business Center, #110
King of Prussia, PA 19406
(610) 992-0020
www.ahta.org
Support and education resource for people interested in horticultural therapy.

Charley's Greenhouse & Garden Supply
17979 State Route 536
Mt. Vernon, WA 98273
(800) 322-4707; (360) 873-8264 (fax)
www.charleysgreenhouse.com
Offers a variety of garden tools that are specially made for those with physical difficulties. Ask for "easier gardening" tools.

Pet Partners
875 124th Ave NE, Suite 101
Bellevue, WA 98005
(425) 679-5500; (425) 679-5539 (fax)
www.petpartners.org
info@petpartners.org
Provides information on the human-animal bond and information on how to obtain a service animal.

Gardenscape Tools
(888) 472-3266
www.gardenscapetools.com
Offers a variety of enabling tools.

National Center of Complementary and Alternative Medicine Clearinghouse
(888) 644-6226 (voice); (866) 464-3615 (TTY)
info@nccam.nih.gov
www.nccam.nih.gov

NCM Consumer Products Division
(800) 821-9319
www.ncmedical.com
Sells garden tools that have special handles.

For more information on garden hints, call your local county office of the **Home Extension Service**.

Contact your local **Humane Society** for information about pet therapy.

If you don't have home access to the Internet, ask your local library or senior center to help you locate any Web site.

For more information on garden hints, call your local county office of the Home **Extension Service**.

Contact your local **Humane Society** for information about pet therapy.

If you don't have home access to the Internet, ask your local library to help you locate any Web site.

Special Challenges

Communication ✍ 252

Speech Problems • Improving the Chance of Being Understood • Sexual Expression

AIDS and the Older Adult ✍ 254

Prevention of AIDS

Depression ✍ 255

Common Fears of a Person with a Chronic Illness • Seasonal Affective Disorder • Dealing with Boredom • Continuing Education • The Internet, Computers, Smartphones • Consumer Fraud and the Lure of Sweepstakes

Pain Management ✍ 262

Types of Pain • Pain Reduction Techniques

Abuse ✍ 265

Dealing with Anger and Elder Abuse • What You Can Do • Signs of Elder Abuse

Transportation and Travel ✍ 269

Transportation • Travel • Travel Emergencies • Travel and Living Wills • Travel Discount Guidelines • Traveling with Medications • Traveling with Your Service Dog

Resources ✍ 276

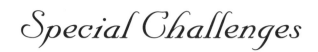

Special Challenges

Communication

Communication is the ability to speak, understand speech, read, write, and gesture. Nonverbal messages are given through silence, body movements, or facial expression. Be aware that words can carry one message, the body another.

Speech Problems

Loss of speech can happen due to damage to the parts of the brain that control language or to lack of oxygen. The person who experiences such a loss still has the same intelligence he or she had before the injury, although this fact may be hard to remember in light of dramatic changes in behavior, which may occur if the loss of speech is the result of stroke or brain injury.

- The communication problem may involve talking or understanding.

- The person may be able to say words at one time and then not at another, or may repeat the same word over and over.

- Left-brain stroke damage affects listening, speaking, reading, and writing.

- Right-brain stroke damage affects non-linguistic skills such as assessing a situation and behaving appropriately, controlling facial expressions, and understanding tones of voice.

A speech therapist can suggest specific tasks to help the person communicate—for example:

- Using pictures instead of words

- Teaching specific exercises to strengthen the muscles of the face, lips, or tongue

To communicate better with the person in your care, try:

- Getting the person's attention by lightly touching her arm before speaking

- Speaking slowly and simply

- Asking questions that require simple yes/no answers

- Providing opportunities for the person to hear speech

- Helping the person communicate frustrations

- Pacing activities, because the person will tire easily

Improving the Chance of Being Understood

When talking to a person with hearing loss follow these guidelines:

- Sit in the light so your lips and facial expressions can be seen.

- Make eye contact.

- Use simple sentences.

- Use body language (nodding, pointing) and lots of facial expression.

- Before starting a conversation, introduce what you are going to talk about ("Mom, let's talk about our vacation"). When you change the subject, say so ("Now, let's talk about dinner").

- Speak louder without shouting. Shouting makes words more difficult to understand.

> **NOTE** If the person in your care has a buzzing in the ear, called tinnitus, ask your health care professional about a tinnitus mask that drowns out the humming with "white noise." A loudly ticking clock or the static of a radio can also create white noise.

Sexual Expression

A disability does not equate with loss of sexual feelings. The needs for intimacy and sharing do not change, although the ability to move in the usual manner may have changed. To improve your spouse's ability to exercise sexual expression, try to increase his or her self-esteem and downplay the role of "patient." Ask your health care professional about assistive devices and techniques for enhanced sexual activities.

AIDS and the Older Adult

AIDS is a disease caused by a virus called HIV. HIV attacks the body's immune system and when the immune system fails, it can no longer fight diseases. People with HIV seem healthy at first. As the disease progresses, they begin to get sicker with infections. When this happens, they are diagnosed with AIDS.

Older people are at risk for AIDS. Symptoms include short-term memory loss; tiredness; experiencing fevers, weight loss, and skin sores; and having swollen lymph glands in the neck. If you suspect AIDS, find a doctor who knows about the latest research by calling your local medical school's department of infectious diseases for a list of experts.

Prevention of AIDS

In older people, sexual activity is the most common cause of HIV infection. The second most common cause is a blood transfusion received before 1985. Since 1985, blood banks have been testing all blood for HIV, so there is little danger of getting HIV from transfusions.

If you are caring for someone with HIV virus or AIDS or if you have the condition, follow some basic rules:

- Always use gloves when providing personal care or handling bodily fluids.

- Always use condoms with penetrative sex.

- Realize that HIV cannot be spread by being coughed or sneezed on by an infected person.

Depression

Aging is a healthy, normal process and not an illness. However, negative emotions and mental attitudes can result in disease. Personality changes with chronic illness can be dramatic, and people with worsening conditions can suffer personality changes that are as permanent as the disease. The most common mental health problems of the aged are depression, anxiety, dementia (e.g., Alzheimer's disease), substance abuse, and paranoia. The suicide rate is higher for the elderly than for any other age group.

Old age is difficult because a person has to make adjustments due to loss of physical strength or health, retirement, death of a spouse, new living arrangements, and the need to accept and prepare for death.

NOTE Depression is often misdiagnosed as dementia or Alzheimer's, but there are differences. Also, several drugs and medical conditions can lead to memory loss. These problems can be reversed, so it is important to get a correct diagnosis for anyone suspected of having Alzheimer's or dementia.

Common Fears of a Person with a Chronic Illness

- Loss of self-image

- Loss of control over life

- Loss of independence and fear of abandonment

- Fear of living alone and being lonely

- Fear of death

You can help deal with these powerful emotions by:

- Pointing out the person's strengths and focusing on small successes

- Restoring areas of control to the person by giving as many choices as possible

- Finding new ways for the person to adjust to limitations

- Providing insight into sources of meaning in life

- Changing your attitude about the person's disability

- Recognizing that humor is healing and providing large doses of laughter to stimulate a positive attitude, providing humorous books, comics, cartoons, television, or movies

- Allowing the person to cry at hearing news of a diagnosis

- Allowing for the power of silence

- Providing opportunities for peer support and friendship (which works exceptionally well with the elderly)

Seasonal Affective Disorder

Some depression can be brought on by the dark, gloomy days of winter. This type of depression may be treated by sitting in front of full-spectrum lights for 1 hour per day. However, be wary of gadgets that promise miraculous results.

Dealing with Boredom

Boredom is another problem for people who are ill, and fighting it can take all your creativity. Try—

- Watching funny movies

- Taking car or bus trips

- Listening to music, especially from the person's youth

- Taking up hobbies

- Going to social events

- Playing board games and card games

- Attending public library discussion events

- Joining local activist organizations like caregiver advocacy, the League of Women Voters, or Gray Panthers. Many have "get involved" links on their Web sites.

- Spending time with others in similar difficulties—in religious groups, recreation centers, stroke clubs (contact the National Stroke Association), or the YMCA/YWCA

- Being involved in volunteer service organizations such as the Retired & Senior Volunteer Program

- Using a computer and accessing sites on the Internet (which helps prevent loneliness through interesting activity and provides the ability to communicate with family and friends through e-mail)

Continuing Education

When time allows, attending continuing education classes at local colleges or correspondence schools can provide education opportunities. There are opportunities for both academic and nonacademic classes (for example, boat building, ceramics, and garden design). Classes offered online for those with time constraints and a home computer are a great value.

To find the program that fits your needs:

- Check college programs in your area.

- Check organizations such as museums, botanical gardens, and arts groups.

- Check Internet listings devoted to distance learning.

- Check PBS Adult Service Online, which offers college courses based on their documentaries.

- Check high school evening courses.

Tip

TUITION DISCOUNTS

Some states are encouraging older students to attend college by offering tuition discounts at public institutions. Adult Education Programs are geared for re-entry students and have lower fees.

The Internet, Computers, Smartphones

By using a computer or smartphone, the Internet provides a simple way for seniors to "surf" the Web or use electronic email to stay in touch with family and friends.

A computer is ideal for the person who has difficulty writing, and it can make life simpler for anyone through these features—

- Enabling a person to type with spell check instead of write letters

- Providing easy duplication of letters by personalizing each letter for the recipient

- Enabling a person to shop via the computer

- Tracking household and investments accounts

- Paying bills through your bank electronically

- Having access to the Internet for information about a limitless array of subjects

Computer software is available that helps users who are visually impaired, deaf, or have other disabilities. One example is Dragon Speech software; you talk, and it types what you say with close accuracy.

> *Tip* **TECHNOLOGY**
> Check the local library for computers-for-seniors classes or for help with locating any Web site. Or, visit your local senior center because many times they offer classes on computer use.

Consumer Fraud and the Lure of Sweepstakes

Lonely elderly people are especially vulnerable to fraudulent telephone solicitations that offer the hope of winning a cash sweepstakes or that appeal to their sense of charity. Some—usually those who are widowed and isolated from their families—even become "addicted" to the attention of telemarketers or "calls for cash" from TV evangelist. Fearful victims are often concerned that their savings will not cover all their living costs and see grand prizes as their only hope.

To help an elderly person avoid becoming a victim of fraud, suggest that certain common-sense rules be followed when receiving calls from telephone solicitors:

- Be wary of a caller who is overly friendly and calls you by your first name.

- Be wary of a caller who insists that you act immediately.

- Be wary of any caller who asks you to send a check by Western Union or overnight delivery.

- Be wary of calls before 8:00 A.M., after 9:00 P.M., or during the weekend.

- Never buy anything by telephone unless you made the contact.

- When construction workers or repairmen are inside your home, remove all personal information from their view.

- Never give out your credit card number unless you have made the contact.

- Never give out your bank account, Social Security, Medicare, or Medicaid number over the telephone or to people you do not know.

- Be wary of anyone pushing you to do something you do not want to do.

- Never contribute to an organization over the telephone, even if you are familiar with the name. Ask the caller to send you a written request.

- If the caller says that phoning saves the charity postage costs, insist the solicitation is sent in writing.

- Be wary of free gifts requiring that you pay shipping charges—your credit card may billed for items you don't want.

- Beware of a request to prepay taxes on a prize. In legitimate awards, the sweepstakes promoter will withhold taxes or report your winnings to the Internal Revenue Service.

- Be wary of securities, investment, or home repair offers that sound too good to be true. Ask for written confirmation of the service or investment opportunity. Consult with a friend or relative before making a decision.

- Do not take money from your bank account if a stranger asks you to—even if he says he is a bank employee and is testing a bank teller.

- Do not allow anyone to send a messenger to your home to pick up a payment.

- Do not fall prey to fraudulent solicitors. JUST HANG UP.

- Never open your door to a stranger, especially if he says it is urgent.

- Check recent known scams and get information on how to avoid becoming a victim by contacting the **National Consumers League** at http://nclnet.org/

- If you continue to receive phone calls from the same company, call your local District Attorney's Office of Consumer Fraud or local police to report the name of the company.

To be removed from national telemarketing *telephone* lists, register every 5 years at www.donotcall.gov (The National Do Not Call Registry by the Federal Trade Commission) where you can also file a complaint or write to:

Telephone Preference Center
Direct Marketing Association
P.O. Box 1559
Carmel, NY 10512

To be removed from national *junk mailing* lists, you must register every 3 years for this service. Here's how:

Register by mail. Send a letter with your name, address and signature along with a $1 processing fee (check or money order made payable to DMA) to:

DMA Mail Prefer-Ence Service
PO Box 643
Carmel, NY 10512

Opt-out of pre-screened *credit offers*. You can substantially reduce the number of pre-screened, pre-approved credit card applications you receive by calling 888-5OPTOUT (888-567-8688), or sign up online at www.optoutprescreen.com

Include your full name and telephone number as well as any variations such as J. Brown, Mrs. James Brown, etc., plus a $1 check or money order. Consider collecting the labels from all junk mail for a few months, taping them to a sheet of paper, mailing it to the service, and requesting that all the listed variations be removed. The service is updated quarterly, so it will take a few months for your request to be processed.

To be taken off the Department of Motor Vehicles mailing list, contact your local DMV office.

> **NOTE** To avoid the chance of theft or misplacement, have monthly pension or Social Security checks deposited directly to the recipient's bank account.

Pain Management

Pain is an individual experience that is tied to both physical and mental states. Even noise makes a person tense, which can contribute to pain. Fatigue, depression, and anxiety can make pain harder to tolerate. (Lying in bed does not lessen the pain, although it may appear that the person is comfortable and relaxed.)

Types of Pain

Pain falls into two categories:

Acute—short-term pain from illness or injury, which can be managed with prescribed narcotics and will subside when the injury heals

Chronic—pain that begins with an illness, is long term (more than 6 months), and is controlled with medications, which may create other problems as the tolerance to those medications increases

Pain can be described as—

- Sharp

- Stabbing

- Hot

- A dull ache

- Constant or intermittent

- Occurring in a specific location and unrelieved by changing position or by rest

- Associated with numbness or extreme weakness

Pain Reduction Techniques

The most effective methods for relieving pain are pain medications (analgesics), sleep, immobilization, and distraction. (Also, heat and cold increase or decrease circulation to the affected area, but should not be used without specific instructions from a doctor.)

To reduce pain, consider:

- Distraction through TV, music, or reading aloud

- Distraction from a medical procedure by massaging the person's hand

- Reduction of stress and promotion of healing through relaxation, meditation, and prayer

 NOTE Although good nutrition will not relieve pain, it promotes healing by strengthening the body.

Pain can be controlled through the following techniques:

- **Acupuncture**—insertion of needles into designated points of the body

- **Acupressure**—pressure and massage at acupuncture points

- **Biofeedback**—the monitoring of reactions to conscious and subconscious thoughts by measuring changes in blood pressure, temperature, and body organs

- **Deep Breathing**—slow deep breaths taken through the nose and exhaled slowly through pursed lips (relieves pain by increasing oxygen to brain)

- **Drugs**—narcotics provide very strong relief but can be addicting if taken long term

- **Hypnosis**—an altered state of consciousness that replaces a focus on pain with attention to another idea

- **Meditation**—a technique for visualizing relief from pain

- **Placebo**—a "sugar" pill that fools the body into thinking it is taking a pain killer and signals pain relief

- **Psychotic Transfer**—a technique that involves having two people go into a meditative state so they can "transfer" pain from one to the other

- **Surgery**—permanent severing of nerves to block pain (a step that requires careful consideration)

- **Topical Pain Relievers**—creams, rubs, or sprays applied to muscles or joints for pain relief in a specific area

- **Transcutaneous Nerve Stimulator (TNS)**—an electronic device placed over acupuncture points

 Sound sleep is often interrupted in older people because of chronic pain and other discomforts. Since a person does not require less sleep as he or she ages, expect more naps during the day.

Abuse

Abusive behavior is never acceptable. Although tensions can mount in the most loving families and result in frustration and anger, an emotionally damaging or physically forceful response is not okay. When this happens, call for a time-out, and call for help.

Physical abuse usually begins in the process of giving or receiving personal help. For instance, the caregiver might be too rough during dressing or grooming, or the care receiver might accidentally scratch the caregiver during a transfer. Once anger and frustration reach this level, abuse by either person may become frequent.

The dangers of physical abuse are easy to see, but emotional abuse is also unhealthy and damaging. Continued shaming, harsh criticism, or controlling behaviors can damage the self-esteem of either person.

Communicating When the Person in Your Care Is Angry

To help defuse a situation so that it doesn't become a problem, here is how to communicate with someone who is angry.

DO

- Be patient, calm, courteous, sympathetic, and show your concern and caring.

- Be open to listening to the person explain the problem before you respond with an answer.

- Look at the problem from the point of view of the person in your care.

- Remember, the person is upset about a situation, not you.

DON'T

- Be defensive and angry.

- Raise your voice (yelling never helps).

- Intimidate the person in your care.

- It is important that you, as caregiver, manage your anger. Ask, "What can we do to make things better?" Think about your own feelings and what button is being pushed. Understanding what is upsetting you will help you from losing control.

Tips You Can Use to Defuse Anger

1. Communicate. Tell the person in your care that you understand or are trying to. "If it happened to me, I'd be angry too."

2. Remind the person that she has choices. Because of her anger she may not realize the choices she has.

3. Affirm her feelings. Say, "I see you are angry."

4. Repeat yourself like a broken record. Softly repeat what is necessary.

NOTE Older people, especially those with dementia, are very sensitive to your mood and body language. Use eye contact, lean forward with interest, and keep a relaxed expression.

What You Can Do

Help the person in your care identify a trusted person who can be called on for help. The Adult Protective Services Agency—a component of the human service agency in most states—is typically responsible for investigating reports of domestic elder abuse and providing help and guidance. Other professionals who may be able to help include doctors or nurses, police officers, lawyers, and social workers.

If you suspect elder abuse in an institutional setting, such as a nursing home, report concerns to your state long-term-care ombudsman.

Each state has such an ombudsman program to investigate and address nursing-home complaints. The **National Center on Elder Abuse** Web site maintains a list of phone numbers, by state, which you can call for assistance if you suspect domestic or institutional elder abuse. Visit http://www.ncea.aoa.gov/. If someone you care about is in imminent danger, call 911 immediately, even if in doubt.

Out-of-State Calls

If your concern is for someone who lives in another state, call the **Family Caregiver Alliance, National Center on Caregiving** at (800) 445-8106 or eldercare Locator [(800) 677-1116] for the in-state phone number. The people who staff the locator can help you to find assistance. All these hotlines are free and anonymous.

Signs of Elder Abuse

Knowing the signs and symptoms of abuse can help you determine if there is a problem.

Signs and symptoms may include:

- Physical injury—bruises, cuts, burns or rope marks, broken bones or sprains that can't be explained.

- Emotional abuse—feeling of helplessness, a hesitation to talk openly, fear, withdrawal, depression, feelings of denial or agitation.

- Lack of physical care—malnourishment, weight loss, poor hygiene, as well as bedsores, soiled bedding, unmet medical needs.

- Unusual behaviors—changes in the person's behavior or emotional state such as withdrawal, duress, fear, or anxiety, apathy.

- Changes in living arrangements.

- Unexplained changes such as the appearance of previously uninvolved relatives or newly met strangers moving in.

- Financial changes—missing money or valuables, unexplained financial transactions, unpaid bills despite available funds, and sudden transfer of assets.

Be alert to the senior's comments about being taken advantage of.

Those most at risk of abuse or neglect are women or those who suffer from dementia. Every year, an estimated 4 million older Americans are victims of physical, psychological, or other forms of abuse and neglect. Those statistics may not tell the whole story. For every case of elder abuse and neglect reported to authorities, experts estimate as many as 23 cases go undetected.
Source: American Psychological Association

Transportation and Travel

Transportation

A network of transportation services, public and private, will pick up the disabled and the elderly at their homes. These services rely on vans and paid drivers and run on a schedule to specific locations. Free transportation is available from community volunteer organizations, although most public services charge on a sliding scale.

 Some states offer transportation to necessary medical care for Medicaid recipients. Check with your local Medicaid office to see if the person in your care qualifies.

Community transportation services resources are provided by:

- Home health care agencies
- Public health departments
- Religious organizations
- Civic clubs
- Local American Red Cross

- Area Agency on Aging
- Local public or private transportation companies

Tip Check out states paratransit resources at:
www.1800taxicab.com/paratransit.htm
Or, call (800) TAX-ICAB for help nationwide.

Travel

Some group tours and cruise lines cater to the elderly or disabled traveler. Before traveling long distances with a person who has a chronic condition, however, consult the person's doctor.

Tip **TRAVEL PLANNING**
If you, as the primary caregiver, are traveling for an extended period, consider investing in a smartphone so you can be reached in case of emergency.

Travel Emergencies

In the event of an emergency abroad, contact American Citizen Services (ACS) in the foreign offices of American consulates and embassies.

American Citizens Services will assist with:

- Lists of doctors, dentists, hospitals, and clinics
- Informing the family if an American becomes ill or injured while traveling
- Helping arrange transportation to the United States on a commercial flight (must be paid by the traveler)

- Explaining various options and costs for return of remains or burial

- Helping locate you, the caregiver, if you are traveling when a family member becomes ill

Travel and Living Wills

If a person becomes disabled with a life-threatening illness while traveling, the medical personnel in foreign countries may not accept the validity of an advance directive (or any other form a personal attorney has drawn up). If a person is traveling and has an illness that requires breathing devices or other life-prolonging treatments, it may be impossible to end the treatment without a medical evacuation back to the United States. However, there a few basic precautions you can take to ensure that a person's wishes are carried out:

- Take a copy of the living will on the trip. Let any other traveling companions know where it is packed.

- Take health-care directive documents with you.

- If traveling in the United States, consider signing the form used in the state where you might be traveling.

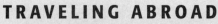

Tip   **TRAVELING ABROAD**
When traveling in tropical countries, use the standard traveler's rule: boil it, peel it, cook it, or forget it!

Travel Discount Guidelines

- The major airlines sell coupon books to those 62 and older.

- Sometimes a caregiver and the traveling companion can get the same discount.

Checklist Travel for the Person with a Chronic Condition

✓ Let the person's primary care doctor know of your travel plans.

✓ Take more of the person's medications than needed, along with a list of names and dosages.

✓ Check with the doctor to see if an immunization against hepatitis A is recommended if traveling to high-risk areas.

✓ Take a list of all medical conditions.

✓ Use a Medic-Alert identification bracelet for the person in care.

✓ Take a copy of his EKG.

✓ Read her insurance policy before taking the trip to see how "emergency" is defined.

✓ If medical care is needed during the trip, get copies of all bills to support claims for reimbursement.

✓ Check into reciprocal agreements between the person's health plan and a provider in the area you will visit.

✓ If you anticipate the need for medical care, call ahead or ask your HMO to help you make doctor's appointments in the new location.

✓ Consider buying traveler's insurance. Study the policy terms regarding pre-existing conditions. READ THE FINE PRINT.

✓ Check that medical equipment is insured for loss or theft.

✓ Consider taking a portable grab bar on the trip.

✓ If traveling to a foreign country, see if the policy allows for medical evacuation.

✓ Take the person's health insurance card and the HMO's toll free number for travelers.

✓ Take copies of the pages in the insurance benefits booklet dealing with emergency access.

✓ Carry a card listing phone numbers of next-of-kin in case of illness during the trip.

✓ Carry a copy of the Consular Information Sheet of the country you are visiting.

✓ Write the primary care doctor's number and beeper number on the health insurance card, along with the date of the last tetanus injection.

✓ If taking a cruise, ask if a doctor with experience in emergency medicine or family practice will be on board.

✓ If the person in your care has a heart condition, check to make sure your airline carries a defibrillator in the event of cardiac arrest. Most major airlines carry them now.

✓ Tell the travel agent or airline that you will require a wheelchair and ask to have your request noted on the ticket.

✓ Call ahead to the airport, bus terminal, or train station to request assistance.

✓ If a flight is delayed for more than four hours, an airline has a duty to provide a meal that is comparable to the meal offered on the flight—if asked for by the passenger.

- The companion can use the discount coupon only on the same itinerary.

- Canadian Association of Retired Persons (A New Vision of Aging for Canada) and American Association of Retired Persons (AARP) members can sometimes get a discount in hotels or retail stores.

- A Medicare card can be used as identification for travel discounts, but it's best to have a state photo ID card or drivers license.

There are all kinds of discounts for seniors. The age often varies as to when you can qualify for a senior discount, but it is usually 50, as it is with AARP members, or sometimes 55 or even 60+. Often, just showing a driver's license or other identification will allow you a senior discount, but many establishments and services ask you to register to get a card identifying you as a senior eligible for any senior discount they offer.

To show the difference in qualifying ages, here are some examples of senior and travel discounts:

- Amtrak Everyday: 15% discount on adult rail fare with some exclusions; for those 62+

- Greyhound: 10% discount for adults 55+

- Best Western: At least 10% off regular room rates for those 55+

- Banana Republic; 10% discount everyday for those 50+

For a list of discounts, visit www.retiredbrains.com and search "Discounts for Seniors".

One common fraud is the offer of a "travel agent" ID card to qualify for discounts through booking your travel. The only card accepted as travel agent identification to qualify for discounts is the International Airlines Travel Agent (IATAN) ID card. Visit www.iatan.org.

Traveling with Medications

Traveling with medications should not stop you and your care receiver from enjoying travel in the United States and abroad. Some tours or cruise lines require a note from the doctor stating that the person is fit to travel. Here are some tips when traveling with medications:

- Bring enough medication to last through your trip plus some extras.

- Pack your meds in a carry-on bag—luggage can stray or become lost.

- Keep all medication in original containers with original prescription labels.

- Make a list of the medications the person takes, and why, with brand and generic names. Make a copy and pack one copy separately.

- Make arrangements for refrigerating the medication.

- If intravenous medication is used, carry a used-needle container.

- Bring the person insurance ID card, plus instructions for accessing a physician where you are going.

- Bring the doctor name and contact information, in case of emergency.

Traveling with Your Service Dog

Have your dog's picture ID card, a doctor note prescribing your animal's service, and a tag or vest for easy identification. If you have further questions about service animals or other requirements of the Americans with Disabilities Act (ADA), call the U.S. Department of Justice's toll-free ADA Information Line at (800) 514-0301 (voice) or (800) 514-0383 (TDD). A revised version of the ADA is available at: http://www.ada.gov/service_animals_2010.htm

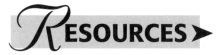

RESOURCES ➤

Abuse

National Center on Elder Abuse (NCEA)
c/o University of California, Irvine
Program in Geriatric Medicine
101 The City Drive South
200 Building
Orange, CA 92868
(855) 500-3537 (ELDR)
(714) 456-7933 (fax)
www.ncea.aoa.gov
Offers fact sheets, reporting numbers, news, publications, and resources.

AIDS Resources

CDC National Prevention Information Network
P.O. Box 6003
Rockville, MD 20849-6003
(800) CDC-INFO (232-4636) (voice)
(888) 232-6348 (TTY)
cdcinfo@cdc.gov

www.cdcnpin.org
Offers free government publications and information about resources on HIV/AIDS, viral hepatitis, sexually transmitted diseases (STDs), and tuberculosis.

National AIDS HOTLINE
(800) 342-AIDS (2437) 24 hours a day, 7 days a week
(800) 344-SIDA (7432) (Spanish) 8 A.M.–2 A.M. EST, 7 days per week
(800) AIDS-889 (243-7889) (TTY) 10 A.M.–10 P.M. EST, M–F
Offers general information and local referrals to support groups for caregivers.

National Institute on Aging
Building 31, Room 5C27
31 Center Drive, MSC 2292
Bethesda, MD 20892
(800) 222-2225
(800) 222-4225 (TTY)
niaic@nia.nih.gov
www.nia.nih.gov
A government program that provides free publications on aging and related health issues.

Social Security Administration
(800) SSA-1213 (772-1213) (voice)
(800) 325-0778 (TTY)
www.ssa.gov

OR

Contact your local Social Security office.
Disability benefit programs that provide financial assistance to eligible AIDS patients.

Disability Benefits 101

http://www.db101.org/

"Disability Benefits 101" gives you tools and information on employment, health coverage, and benefits, so you can plan ahead and learn how work and benefits go together.

Depression/Continuing Education Resources

Administration on Aging

www.aoa.gov

An information "ferret" with links to the Administration on Aging, Social Security Administration, National Institute of Health, and more.

American Speech-Language-Hearing Association

2200 Research Boulevard
Rockville, MD 20850-3289
(800) 638-8255
(301) 296-5700 (in Maryland)
(301) 296-5650 (TTY)
www.asha.org

Provides free information on various communication disorders and makes referrals to audiologists and speech pathologists.

University of Wisconsin Independent Learning

https://il.wisconsin.edu/index.aspx

OR

University of Wisconsin System eCampus

http://www.ecampus.wisconsin.edu/

Council of Better Business Bureaus

(703) 276-0100
www.bbb.org

Will refer you to the Council of Better Business Bureaus in your area, by zip code, for the business you are inquiring about.

Education Index
www.educationindex.com

Healthy.net
www.healthy.net
Web site with an orientation toward homeopathic, holistic health and other alternative medicines.

Museums of the USA
www.museumca.org/usa

National Organization for Victim Assistance (NOVA)
510 King Street, Suite 424
Alexandria, VA 22314
(800) 879-6682 (TRY-NOVA) 9 A.M.–5 P.M. EST, M–F
(703) 535-5500 (fax)
www.trynova.org
A nonprofit organization that provides the name and number of a victim's assistance support group in your area. They also provide training in crisis response.

PBS Adult Learning Service Online
http://www.pbslearningmedia.org/
http://www.aetn.org/education/adulted/aboutpbsliteracylink

SeniorNet
PBS Adult Learning Service Online
http://www.pbslearningmedia.org/
http://www.aetn.org/education/adulted/aboutpbsliteracylink
www.seniornet.org
An educational nonprofit organization with links to other online sources for older adults in the areas of government, learning, health, wellness, and other areas of interest. SeniorNet operates learning centers where seniors are taught computer skills and learn programs to access the Internet.

Pain Management Resources

American Academy of Medical Acupuncture
1970 E. Grand Avenue, Suite 330
El Segundo, CA 90245
(310) 364-0193
www.medicalacupuncture.org
Will provide the names of member acupuncturists who are also medical doctors.

Pain Connection
Chronic Pain Outreach Center, Inc.
12320 Parklawn Drive
Rockville, MD 20852
(301) 231-0008
(301) 231-6668 (fax)
www.painconnection.org
Offers support groups, specialized classes, and many other resources and materials to empowering people with chronic pain.

The Worldwide Congress on Pain
http://www.pain.com

Transportation and Travel Resources

Centers for Disease Control and Prevention
1600 Clifton Road
Atlanta, GA 30333
(800) CDC-INFO (232-4636)
(888) 232-6348 (TTY)
cdc-info@cdc.gov
www.cdc.gov
Provides recommendations on vaccinations and health data for travel to specific countries; also provides information about diseases such as malaria and yellow fever.

Consular Information Program
Bureau of Consular Affairs
State Department
(202) 647-3000 (automatic fax)
(202) 647-5225 (recorded messages)
www.travel.state.gov
Provides travel advisory information and emergency assistance. From the Web site, you can read or print Tips for Traveling Abroad, including "Medical Information for Americans Abroad."

Travel Assistance International
Corporate Offices:
PO Box 668
Millersville, MD 21108
(410) 987-6233
Claims Administration:
Seven Corners, Inc
303 Congressional Blvd.
Carmel, IN 46032
(800) 335-0477
(317) 575-2652
(317)-575-2256 (fax)

Assistance Center: (800) 643-5525
Outside North America, call collect: (317) 818-2098
http://travelassistanceinternational.com
A for-profit company that provides members with worldwide, 24/7 comprehensive travel services such as on-site emergency medical payments, emergency medical transportation, and assistance with medication replacement.

CARP A New Vision of Aging for Canada
http://www.carp.ca/

Lesbian Gay Bisexual Transgendered (LGBT)

Services & Advocacy for Gay, Lesbian, Bisexual & Transgender Elders (SAGE)
305 7th Avenue 15th Floor
New York, NY 10001
(212) 741-2247
(212) 366-1947
info@sageusa.org
www.sageusa.org
Provides resources for LGBT people age 50 and older, including HIV/AIDS information and referrals.

If you don't have home access to the Internet, ask your local library or senior center to help you locate any Web site.

Diet, Nutrition, and Exercise

Diet, Nutrition, and Exercise

A person's quality of life can often be improved by focusing on those aspects of health that can be changed. Good health has a lot to do with what you do each and every day. Eating right and being physically active are areas in which you can be in control. The lifestyle habits you choose can have a lot to do with feeling good today and staying healthy tomorrow.

Proper nutrition is basic to good health. An older person's diet should avoid high-calorie, low-nutrient food. As the body ages, a person has to make more of an effort to eat wisely. However, there is no need to change food habits to drastically lower fat intake.

Most older people need fewer calories to maintain normal body weight. Their bodies absorb fewer nutrients so they must eat high-nutrient food to maintain good health. They must get more nutrients from less food. If a person does not get enough calories, the body will use stored nutrients for energy. When this happens, the person becomes weaker and is more likely to get infections.

Check with the doctor before starting any special diets, especially for the person with a swallowing impairment. Also, check with a doctor, pharmacist, or registered dietitian to know what effect prescription medicines have on nutritional needs.

NOTE Use every means possible to perk up the appetite. Make sure the person's dentures fit correctly and that his or her glasses are adequate. We eat with our eyes before we ever touch our food.

Careful Food Preparation

Older people are especially susceptible to illness from unsafe food, so be extra careful when preparing their meals.

- Wash your own hands and the hands of the person in your care with antibacterial soap before preparing or serving food.

- Dry hands with a paper towel.

- Disinfect the sink and kitchen counters with a solution of 1 teaspoon chlorine bleach per liter of water. (Save the solution for just one week because it loses strength.)

- Air drying dishes is more sanitary than using a dish towel.

- Check expiration dates carefully, and discard all meats that are past the expiration date on the label.

- Cook all red meat and fish thoroughly.

- Cook hamburgers or chopped meat to an internal temperature of 160° F. (There is much less chance of being infected by a solid piece of meat like a steak or roast because bacteria collects only on the outside of those cuts.)

- Cook meat to at least at an oven temperature of 300° F.

NOTE If the pathogens are present when meat is ground, more of the meat surface is exposed to the harmful bacteria. Grinding mixes the bacteria throughout the meat. Bacteria multiply rapidly in the "Danger Zone," where temperatures are between 40°F and 140°F (4.4°C and 60°C). To keep bacteria levels low, store ground beef at 40°F (4.4°C) or colder and use within 2 days, or freeze it. To destroy harmful bacteria, cook ground beef to a safe minimum internal temperature of 160°F (71.1°C). Source: USDA

- Keep hot foods hot at or above 140°F or more and cold foods below 40°F or colder.

- Keep the refrigerator between 35 and 40F°.

- Cook eggs until the yolks are no longer runny.

- Don't serve raw eggs in milk shakes or other drinks.

- Don't serve oysters, clams, or shellfish raw.

- Wash all fruits and vegetables thoroughly.

- Avoid unpasteurized milk and cider.

NOTE If the water temperature is set too low, the dishwasher will not sterilize the dishes.

Nutrition Guidelines for the Elderly

Be aware of any medical condition that would require restrictions such as salt (congestive heart failure) or potassium (kidney failure).

- Make tasty, nutritionally well-balanced meals that promote good bowel function and a normal flow of urine.

- Offer drinking water or liquids at mealtime to make chewing and swallowing easier.

- Avoid lard, bacon fat, coconut and palm kernel oil, sweets, and highly seasoned foods.

- Serve fresh fruits and vegetables. They are good sources of fiber and Vitamins A and C and they prevent constipation.

- Do not serve too much refined food, which lacks fiber and contributes to constipation.

- To improve sluggish appetites, use seasonings like herbs, spices, lemon juice, peppers, garlic, and vinegar, especially if salt is restricted.

Boosting Calorie or Protein Intake

- Offer most of the food when the person is most hungry.

- Encourage the person to eat food with the fingers if it increases intake.

- Add non-fat powdered milk to any food with liquid in it, such as desserts, soups, gravy, and cereal.

- Add butter, whipped cream, or sour cream to foods.

- Add cottage cheese or ricotta cheese to casseroles, scrambled eggs, and desserts.

- Grate hard cheeses on bread, meats, vegetables, eggs, and casseroles.

- Use instant breakfast powder in milk drinks and desserts.

- Add nuts, seeds, and wheat germ to breads, cereal, casseroles, and desserts.

- Add beaten eggs to mashed potatoes, sauces, vegetable purees, and cooked puddings.

- Add honey, jam, or sugar to bread, milk drinks, fruit, and yogurt desserts.

- Add mayonnaise to salads and sandwiches.

Quick and Easy Snacks

Be sure to first check with your doctor about sugar, salt, or potassium restrictions.

- Buttered popcorn

- Cheese on crackers

- Chocolate milk

- Fruits, especially ripe bananas

- Granola cookies

- Hard-boiled eggs

- Milkshakes

- Puddings

- Raisins, nuts, prunes

- Yogurt

PREPARING FOOD

When preparing a meal for the person in your care, put a small amount in the blender to make it easier for the person in your care to eat.

Therapeutic Diets

Keep the doctor informed about the diet you follow. A special diet may be prescribed to:

- Improve or maintain a person's health

- Change the amount of bulk, as in a high fiber diet

- Change the consistency of food, as in a special soft diet

- Eliminate or decrease certain foods

- Change the number of calories

Dehydration Prevention

As a person ages, he feels less thirsty, so a special effort should be made to provide enough fluids. A person's fluid balance can be affected by medication, emotional stress, exercise, nourishment, general health, and the weather. Dehydration, especially in the elderly, can increase confusion and muscle weakness and cause nausea. Nausea, in turn, will prevent the person from wanting to eat, thereby causing more dehydration.

Preventive Measures Include:

- Encouraging the person to drink 6–8 cups of liquid every day (or an amount determined by the doctor)

- Serving beverages at room temperature

- Providing foods high in liquid (for example, watermelon)

- Avoiding caffeine, which causes frequent urination and dehydration (ask your doctor)

Osteoporosis Prevention

Older people—especially women—often suffer from osteoporosis, a condition that occurs when there is not enough calcium and vitamin D in the diet. Getting lots of calcium and vitamin D is especially important for women in the first few years after menopause, when bone mass is lost more rapidly.

Osteoporosis can be prevented by:

- Getting adequate vitamin D from sunshine a few times per week, and from fortified milk, fatty fish, or a vitamin supplement.

- Getting calcium from dairy foods, leafy vegetables such as kale and collards, broccoli, salmon, and sardines

- Taking calcium supplements. Always take calcium with vitamin D because vitamin D is necessary for the body to absorb calcium. Take the supplements in the evening because calcium is absorbed during sleep.

Between the ages of 51 and 57, it is recommended that people get between 1,000 and 1,200 milligrams of calcium daily to slow bone loss. The recommended amount of vitamin D is 600 milligrams a day.

Recommended Daily Allowances for a Person Over Age 51

If you are concerned that an elderly person is malnourished or gaining weight, do a calorie check periodically. Recommended daily allowances are for people 51 and older are listed here. These are average calorie amounts that are based on the person's activity level:

Women: sedentary – 1,600 calories
      moderately active – 1,800 calories

Men: sedentary – 2,000 calories
     moderately active – 2,200 calories

Because a person's metabolism (how fast they burn up calories) is reduced with aging, older people generally need fewer calories than do young people. Source: USDA

Additional Sources of Calcium, Folate, and Protein

The diets of the elderly are often deficient in these nutrients which are found in the following foods: (* denotes most concentrated sources)

Calcium (one cup serving, except where noted)
    Cheddar cheese (1 oz.)
    Collards (1/2 cup, cooked)
    Lactaid milk, nonfat, calcium fortified*
    Milk, skim or 1%
    Orange juice, with added calcium*
    Ricotta, fat-free (1/4 cup)
    Swiss cheese (1 oz.)*

Total® brand cereal (3/4 cup)*
Yogurt, nonfat, plain*

Folate (one cup serving, except where noted)
Brewer's yeast (1 tablespoon)
Chickpeas or pinto beans, cooked
Ensure brand nutrition supplement
Lentils, cooked*
Orange juice
Product 19 brand cereal*
Red kidney beans
Spinach (1/2 cup, cooked)
Total® brand cereal (3/4 cup)*

Protein (4 oz. serving, except where noted)
Beans or peas (1 cup)
Beef steak, eye of round, well trimmed*
Chicken (without skin or bone)*
Chili with beans (1 cup)
Eggs
Flounder*
Lamb, well trimmed*
Lentils (1 cup cooked)*
Pork tenderloin, well trimmed*
Salmon, canned, drained
Tuna, canned in water, drained*
Turkey (without skin or bone)*
Yogurt, nonfat, plain (8 oz.)

NOTE These may not be the best foods for a person under special medical treatment. Special diets and products to improve nutrition should only be used on the advice of a doctor or registered dietitian. If a special diet is needed due to an existing medical condition or disease, contact your local out-patient dietitian or diabetes treatment program.

Checklist **Nutrition Assessment**

To assess nutrition risk for the person in your care, check the following questions. If the answer to most of the points is Yes, then the person is at risk and you need to contact the doctor for a diet. Answer the questions every six months or whenever you notice big changes in weight or eating habits.

✓ Has she recently lost weight? _____ About how much? _____ lbs.

✓ Has she had any recent appetite loss? _____ For how long? _____ (days, weeks, months)

✓ Does she have difficulty chewing? _____

✓ Does she have difficulty swallowing? _____

✓ Food allergies? _____
_____

✓ A special diet? _____
_____

✓ Have you been given instructions about her diet? _____

✓ Does she eat fewer than 2 meals per day? _____

✓ Does she eat few fruits, vegetables, and dairy products? _____

✓ How many servings per day?
Fruits _____
Vegetables _____
Dairy _____

✓ Does she drink more than 3 alcoholic beverages per day? _____

✓ Does she eat most of her meals alone? _____
_____

Weight Loss

This is not a diet book, but if you or your care receiver are overweight, then losing weight will require some change in diet. Whatever diet your doctor recommends, losing weight is a matter of taking in fewer calories than your body burns. It's like balancing a caloric checkbook, where calories are cash and weight is savings.

Gaining weight – You have a "caloric excess." You are eating more calories than your body is using. You will store these excess calories as fat.

Losing weight – You have a "caloric deficit." You are eating fewer calories than you are using, and your body is drawing on its fat storage cells for energy.

The goal is to be "in balance." You are eating closely the same number of calories that your body is using.

A smartphone with the right app can be a great tool for tracking weight and fitness. One such tool is the Fitbit wristband. It is a device that you can wear all the time. Once you enter your information, it tracks steps, distance, and calories burned, or tracks weight, types of foods, and water intake. During the night, it tracks your sleep quality and wakes you silently in the morning. The Fitbit syncs your data wirelessly to your computer, smartphone, or other device.

NOTE If you eat approximately 10 calories more than you burn every day for a year, you'll gain 1 lb (3,600 calories = 1 lb.).

If you do that for 20 years—just 10 calories more a day—at the end of 20 years, you'll have gained 20 lbs.

Ten calories is an insignificant amount of food. But many people eat hundreds of calories more than they need every day. This simple equation may explain why, of Americans aged 20 and older, 154.7 million are overweight (with a body mass index [BMI] of 25.0 kg/m^2 and higher). Of these, 78.4 million are obese (with a BMI of 30.0 kg/m^2 or more). (American Heart Association/ Stroke Association (2013)

Diet and Nutrition Education

If you need reliable, well-organized, user-friendly advice about a healthy diet, get a copy of *The No-Fad Diet* from the American Heart Association (AHA). It is the only diet book the AHA has ever written, and it contains all the information you need about diet, exercise, and behavior change. It also contains sample meal plans, easy-to-prepare recipes, and information on starting an exercise program. One of the key features of the book is that it addresses the psychological component of changing behavior. The book is available at the American Stroke Association Web site, through online booksellers, or your local bookstore. In addition, AHA offers many cookbooks, all designed to combat cardiovascular disease and stroke.

Cholesterol

Cholesterol is present in the cell wall of every cell in animal bodies, including human animals. The amount of cholesterol determines how permeable (leaky) the cell is. Cholesterol has a couple of other positive roles, but that cell-wall function is the main one. Cholesterol is so important to our basic biology that our bodies manufacture all the cholesterol they need from saturated fat. Dietary cholesterol is extra.

NOTE ▷ Cholesterol manufacture is under genetic control, and it is possible that diet and exercise won't be enough to lower your care receiver's numbers. Cholesterol-lowering medication may be called for. Older cholesterol drugs work to block absorption of dietary cholesterol. A new type of drug addresses the manufacture of cholesterol in the liver.

Tip

Lowering the intake of *saturated fat* will help lower cholesterol level.

Saturated fat is fat that is solid at room temperature, like butter or the fat on meat.

Unsaturated fat is liquid at room temperature, like vegetable oil.

To get from your liver to your cells, cholesterol has to travel in your blood. Although technically a kind of fat, cholesterol is like a wax, think egg-yolk residue on a plate after breakfast. Since blood is mostly water, it doesn't know what to do with wax. It can't dissolve it, so it wraps it in protein. That's where cholesterol gets its other name—lipoprotein.

> **Tip**
>
> Baffled by the LDL/HDL distinction? Low-density lipoprotein (LDL) is *bad* cholesterol, think L for "lousy." Another easy way to remember this is to think of LDL as "less-desirable lipids." LDL cholesterol doesn't move in liquid as well and tends to be stickier and so sticks to blood- vessel walls. High-density lipoprotein (HDL) is the *good* kind, think H for "healthy" or HDL as "highly desirable lipids." HDL tends to flow more freely in the blood stream and is not as sticky.
>
> Whether cholesterol is LDL or HDL is largely determined by activity levels—in other words, you can't eat more or less of either one. To increase HDL levels exercise more.

To reduce the dietary cholesterol of the person in your care you must alter his or her intake of animal products. All meat, dairy, and eggs contain some cholesterol, no matter their fat content, because *all* animal cells contain cholesterol. In addition, tropical oils (palm and coconut) and partially hydrogenated oils also contribute to cholesterol numbers.

> **Tip**
>
> Partially hydrogenated oil is vegetable oil with hydrogen whipped into it, generally to increase shelf life. Nutritionists now label these oils as "trans-fat." It is suspected that trans-fats also contribute to atherosclerosis (a disease in which cholesterol deposits form on the walls of arteries, narrowing them).

Blood Pressure

Diet affects blood pressure because it affects weight, sodium, and atherosclerosis. Atherosclerosis increases blood pressure by narrowing arteries from the inside. Sodium causes water retention because our kidneys need water to maintain a proper electrolyte balance. This retained water puts pressure on the blood vessels and keeps them from relaxing, thereby increasing blood pressure.

Nutrition scientists have formulated the DASH Diet. (DASH stands for Dietary Approach to Stop Hypertension.) The DASH Diet was designed by the National Heart, Lung and Blood Institute after rigorous investigation into which vitamins, minerals, and micronutrients affected blood pressure. (http://dashdiet.org/)

The DASH Diet is low in saturated fat, cholesterol, and total fat. It emphasizes fruits, vegetables, and low-fat dairy foods, and includes whole-grain products, fish, poultry, and nuts. It is reduced in red meat, sweets, and sugar-containing beverages, and is rich in magnesium, potassium, and calcium, as well as protein and fiber. It controls for sodium. Research has reported reductions in blood pressure in as little as two weeks after beginning the DASH diet.

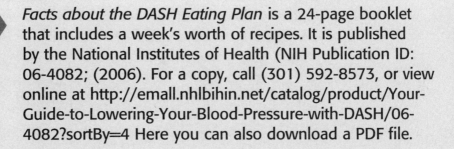

NOTE *Facts about the DASH Eating Plan* is a 24-page booklet that includes a week's worth of recipes. It is published by the National Institutes of Health (NIH Publication ID: 06-4082; (2006). For a copy, call (301) 592-8573, or view online at http://emall.nhlbihin.net/catalog/product/Your-Guide-to-Lowering-Your-Blood-Pressure-with-DASH/06-4082?sortBy=4 Here you can also download a PDF file.

Tip

Blood pressure is affected by more than one biological/chemical mechanism. In order to control high blood pressure, doctors may prescribe more than one blood pressure medication because different drugs work with different mechanisms. Each medication plays a role in reducing the numbers, as does your diet.

A Foundation of Good Nutrition

Bringing good nutrition to the table takes planning, attention, and some imagination. A foundation to healthy eating can be found in the U.S. Department of Agriculture's *MyPyramid*. Making smart choices from each part of the pyramid is the best way to ensure one's body gets the balanced nutrition it needs. Here are some easy tips to make the most of every food group, and get the most from the calories eaten:

- **Focus on fruits.** Select fresh, frozen, canned, or dried over juices for most of your fruit choices.

- **Vary your vegetables.** Choose from a rainbow of colors—dark green, such as broccoli, kale, and spinach; orange, such as carrots, pumpkin, and sweet potatoes; yellow, such as yellow peppers and butternut squash.

- **Make half your grains whole.** When selecting cereals, breads, crackers, or pastas, look to see that the grains listed on the ingredient list are "whole." Whole grains provide a great source of fiber and can help in managing weight and controlling constipation.

- **Keep it lean.** Choose lean meats, fish, and poultry and bake, broil, or grill whenever possible. Try to vary your protein choices and add or substitute beans, peas, lentils, nuts, and seeds to what you eat.

- **Calcium counts.** Include 3 cups of low-fat or fat-free milk, yogurt, or equivalent of low-fat cheeses every day to maintain good bone health. Calcium-fortified foods and beverages can help fill the gap if you don't or can't consume milk.

- **Limit your fat, sugar, and salt.** These "extras" can add up! Check out the nutrition label on foods and look for foods low in saturated and trans fats. Sugars often only provide added calories with little added nutritional value. Choose and prepare foods with little salt or sodium.

Meeting the Challenges of Changing a Diet

Good nutrition is the goal, but food is not just about nutrition. It is about emotions, culture, and being social. What and how we eat is so personal that changing eating habits can be difficult. Special diets and drastic fitness programs sometimes promise the quick fix, or even the cure. Yet, the best advice for care receivers is the same as for everyone: Eat a low-fat diet with a variety of grains, vegetables, and fruits, along with some high-protein foods like meat or dairy products; and balance how many calories you take in with physical activity.

Deciding to change is the first step. But the changes don't have to take place overnight. Start with the easy ones. Then, one by one, add more kinds of vegetables, reduce portion sizes, start eating more low-fat foods.

Here's a checklist for you and the person in your care:

- Be realistic. Make small changes over time. Small steps can work better than giant leaps.

- Be daring and try new foods.

- Be flexible. Balance food intake with physical activity over several days. Don't focus on just one meal or one day.

- Be sensible and practice not overdoing it.

- Be active and choose activities that you enjoy and that fit into the rest of your life.

Special Needs and Considerations

Good nutrition is necessary for everyone, but sometimes things can get in the way of eating right. Ask the nurse, doctor, or pharmacist if any of the medications the person in your care is taking have possible side effects that can interfere with appetite or affect the absorption of important vitamins and minerals.

NOTE Blood Thinner Pills: Your Guide to Using Them Safely
The Agency for Healthcare Research and Quality offers a free booklet and a video about blood thinner medicines. *Staying Active and Healthy with Blood Thinners,* a 10-minute video, features easy-to-understand explanations of how blood thinners work and why it's important to take them correctly. *Blood Thinner Pills: Your Guide to Using Them Safely,* a 24-page booklet, explains how these pills can help prevent dangerous blood clots from forming and what to expect when taking these medicines.

To get a copy of this free booklet and to watch the video, go to http://www.ahrq.gov/patients-consumers/diagnosis-treatment/treatments/btpills/index.html

Here are some tips to ensure that the person in your care gets the nutrition he or she needs.

- The thought of three big meals may be too much for the person. In fact, five to six smaller mini-meals throughout the day may be easier to manage and help keep energy levels high. Keep the fridge and pantry filled with items that provide the nutrition the person in your care needs for good health and watch those that provide little to the diet except calories. Some healthful choices can include reduced-fat cheese sticks, nuts and nut butter, fresh or dried fruit, hardboiled eggs, low-fat yogurt or cottage cheese, bagged salads, and cut raw vegetables.

- Keep meal preparation simple. Focus on one part of the meal, like the main dish and rely on quick-cooking grains, easy-to-heat veggies and a whole-grain roll for side dishes. Save energy by collecting all the ingredients and cooking utensils first and sit down at the counter or table to put it all together.

- When you cook, try to make more than is needed for one meal. Store or freeze the rest in oven-or microwave-ready containers for quick reheating.

- Make the most of the freezer. Stock up on low-fat dinners that can be quickly reheated.

- Save menus from places that deliver healthful meals.

NOTE **Changes in mobility.** If eating habits remain the same while activity drops off, **weight gain** can result. Added weight can increase fatigue, further limit mobility, put a strain on the respiratory and circulatory systems (lungs, heart, blood, blood vessels), and increase the risk of other chronic illnesses. Ask a registered dietitian to recommend an ideal weight and reasonable daily calorie intake to maintain that weight. To get weight under control, pair exercise with healthy eating.

Additionally, inadequate physical activity, lack of weight-bearing exercise, and an increasingly sedentary lifestyle can result from changes in mobility that can contribute to the risk of developing **osteoporosis** (see p. 289)—a condition where bones can become thin and fragile. While building strong bones started early in childhood, keeping them healthy as we grow older requires attention and care. Good nutrition—particularly daily sources of calcium—is important for maintaining bone health.

- Choose nonfat or low-fat dairy products often.

- Eat any type of fish with edible bones, such as canned salmon or sardines.

- Choose dark-green vegetables like kale, broccoli, turnip greens, and mustard greens. The calcium in these veggies is better absorbed than the calcium found in spinach, rhubarb, beet greens, and almonds.

- Calcium-fortified tofu, soy milk, orange juice, breads, and cereals are excellent staples. Check the food labels to see just how much calcium has been added.

- Vitamin D also plays an important role in bone health by helping with the calcium absorption. Our bodies can make vitamin D with just 15–20 minutes of skin exposure to the sun each day. Vitamin D can also be found fortified in foods that contain calcium. Be careful with supplementation because vitamin D is stored in the body and can be toxic in relatively low amounts (>2,000 i.u./day)

NOTE ▶ **Eating and emotions.** Depression can affect people's appetite in different ways. Many people turn to certain foods for comfort when they are depressed. These may be old favorites from childhood—a scoop of mashed potatoes, macaroni and cheese, a bowl of rice pudding. The danger is in overdoing it. These foods are often high in fat, sugar, and calories that can easily add up. On the other hand, some people lose their appetite when they are depressed. Eating with others can help you and the person in your care stay connected. Remember also that being physically active can help decrease the symptoms of depression.

NOTE ▶ **Bladder problems are another issue.** Quite often, fear of having to go to the bathroom frequently or loss of bladder control causes a person to limit fluids. This can cause other problems such as dehydration, dry mouth, difficulty swallowing, loss of appetite, and constipation. Find ways to fit in fluids.

- Take water breaks during the day.

- Have a beverage with meals.

- "Water down" your meals and snacks.

- Take a drink when you pass a water fountain.

- Travel with your own personal supply of bottled water.

> **NOTE** **Bowel management** often involves preventing constipation. Fiber counts—add it up. Fiber is found in cereal, grains, nuts, seeds, vegetables, and fruit. It is not completely digested (broken down) or absorbed (taken in) by the body. A diet rich in fiber (about 25 to 30 grams each day) along with adequate fluid intake and physical activity can help promote good bowel function. Fiber can also provide a sense of fullness, which helps in managing how much one eats.

Exercise as Part of Life

Physical activity and good nutrition are perfect partners in good health. This winning combination finds a balance between what one eats and one's daily activities. Together they help in managing weight and providing energy. Physical activity not only burns calories, but it can also help the person in your care by doing the following:

- Make the most of muscle strength, or even build strength, depending on the program

- Slowly increase the ability to do more for longer periods of time

- Increase range of motion and joint flexibility (the ability to move easily)

- Strengthen the heart

- Decrease feelings of fatigue

- Decrease symptoms of depression

- Maintain regular bowel and bladder functions

- Cut down on the risk of skin breakdown and irritation

- Protect weight-bearing bone mass (spine, hips, legs)

Good physical fitness is made up of three types of exercise: stretching, strengthening, and aerobics. Each is important by itself, but together they can help the person in your care remain active as long as possible. This will help the person deal better with the changes illness may bring.

A person should always stretch before exercise. This warms the muscles, helps prevent stiffness, and improves flexibility and balance. The person should work at his or her own pace, even if it seems very slow. Encourage the person in your care, even if the exercises seem difficult at first. Watch for signs of fatigue. Always cool down after exercise.

Stretching

Regular *s-t-r-e-t-c-h-i-n-g* is the first step, and it can be one of the most enjoyable. Stretching helps muscle rigidity (stiffness). It also helps muscles and joints stay flexible (able to bend). People who are more flexible have an easier time with everyday movement.

Stretching increases range of motion of joints and helps with good posture. It protects against muscle strains or sprains, improves circulation, and releases muscle tension.

Do's and Don'ts of Stretching

- **DO** stretch to the point of a gentle pull.

- **DON'T** stretch to the point of pain.

- **DON'T** bounce while stretching.

- **DON'T** hold the breath during a stretch. Breathe evenly in and out during each stretch.

- **DON'T** compare yourself to others.

Stretching can be done at any time. The person in your care can start the day by stretching before getting out of bed. Have the person stretch throughout the day, while watching television or riding in a car.

Aerobic activities raise the heart rate and breathing, and promote cardiovascular (heart and lung) fitness. Other activities develop strength and flexibility. For example, lifting weights develops strength and can help maintain good bone health. Activities like yoga and gentle stretching can improve flexibility.

Some key points to remember:

- You and the person in your care should talk with the doctor about exercise, target weight, and special needs. If possible, get a referral to a physical therapist to help begin the program.

- An exercise program needs to match the abilities and limitations of the individual. A physical therapist can design a well-balanced exercise program for those who need more help. With some changes, people at all levels of disability can enjoy the benefits of exercise.

- The person in your care should commit to doing what he or she can do on a consistent basis. Choosing activities you both enjoy will help you stick to your fitness plan.

- Start slowly. If the person in your care hasn't been active, begin at a low level of intensity for short periods. Alternate brief periods of exercise with periods of rest until the person in your care begins to build up endurance. Gradually increase how hard you are exercising and the length of time you are doing it.

- Join a group! Exercising with others may give you the motivation and support to keep going.

Get Moving

In addition to a diet prescription, the person in your care may have gotten an exercise prescription. It is important that care receivers participate in some form of calorie-burning activity if at all possible.

> **NOTE** A person begins to get aerobic benefit from exercise when his or her heart rate hits 50 percent of its maximum. No one should exceed 80 percent of his or her maximum heart rate during exercise.
>
> To figure maximum heart rate, subtract age from 220. For example, maximum heart rate for a 60-year-old person is 160. For aerobic benefit, he must get the heart rate up to 80 beats per minute and should not exceed 130 beats per minute.

For many care receivers, because of age or level of debility, the standard exercise prescription of 30 minutes most days of the week is simply not possible. So understand from the beginning that the care receiver's activity level won't look like an active person's.

In Water

Water therapy is a time-tested form of healing. It is also a safe way for a person with a disability and the elderly to exercise because there is no danger of falling. Floating in water allows easy movement and little strain on joints and muscles.

For those who have some weakness on one side of the body, water exercises are a good alternative because the affected side floats and feels lighter in water. Using a kickboard or simply walking in place in water may produce aerobic benefit. Water also resists movement so it produces increased heart rate in less time. Water can also be a good place to exercise for those with balance problems. Talk to a physical therapist about whether a water aerobics class might be appropriate for the person in your care.

Tip

YMCAs often offer water aerobics classes that your care receiver might participate in, as do Easter Seals, community clubs, or community recreation centers.

On Land

Aerobic exercise on land for the elderly or people with disabilities is more problematic. A readily available option is chair exercises. These allow the person to remain seated while providing aerobic benefit.

Tip

Several DVD and video products offer complete workouts, as do some TV programs. In your search engine, type "chair exercises" or "chair dancing" or "workout," or "fitness."

Another option for those with one-sided weakness or even paralysis, is an exercise machine called a seated stepper. These machines allow one to sit upright and move both legs and arms. (Moving arms and legs simultaneously is the most efficient way to increase heart rate and burn calories.) When seated, people don't have to worry about balance, as they would on a stationary bike, stair stepper, or treadmill. The feet are held in place by Velcro straps, so even if one leg is affected, the person can still use the machine. A weak hand can be Velcro-wrapped to one of the arm poles so that it moves back and forth.

Weight Training

Muscles often weaken as a result of not being used. Weight training can be a major help in restoring these muscles. Recent research indicates that targeted strength training in patients with muscle weakness significantly increased muscle power without any negative effects.

Do not take the person in your care to the weight room and just leave her there. She will need supervision and instruction. Most physical trainers do not have enough special training to work with people with disabilities, but increasingly it is possible to find special needs strength trainers who may be able to help. For a basic special needs weight workout, visit **http://www.ilru.org/html/ publications/directory/index.html** for a resource in your area. Also, ask at your community college if they have a Disabled Student Program (DSP) that offers weight training or swimming for special needs individuals.

Fear of Falling

Balance can be affected in a person with a disability, as with stroke, for example, and consequently many elderly people fear falling, with good reason. If the person in your care has balance problems, dizziness, or a spinning sensation, see if you can get a therapy prescription from your doctor.

To reduce fear of falling, therapists often have people practice getting up from a lying position. This increases confidence that they can get up if they fall.

> *Tip*
>
> To improve balance at home, bring a chair to the corner of a room. While the care receiver stands in the corner, she can hold on to the back of the chair and practice moving shoulders and hips together from side to side and then forward and backward.

Remember, before starting any type of workout routine, get advice from your physician. Start slowly with only moderate effort. Give the care receiver time to build strength and stamina. Any amount of exercise helps reduce risk, and the benefits of exercise are cumulative, so find a way to make it easy to get exercise, that way the survivor is more likely to do it. Exercise is a particularly effective way to reduce depression.

And finally, everything said here about the benefits of aerobic exercise and weight training also applies to the caregiver. *You* need exercise as much as the person in your care. Find a way to make it part of most days.

Motivation

Motivation is the #1 factor determining whether people change their lifestyles or fail to follow their exercise and diet prescriptions. While motivation is an inside job, the caregiver has a part to play. Do what you can to make exercise fun. Make the new diet an experiment. If you make either diet or exercise too important, any failure becomes that much more significant. Keep it light hearted, maintain a sense of humor, and join in as much as possible.

No single day of exercise or eating right makes much of a difference in your or your care receiver's health, but 30 days do. Sixty days makes even more of an impact; a year's worth of a new lifestyle will provide remarkable shifts of biomarkers (a specific physical trait used to measure the effects or progress of a disease or condition; thinning hair is an example of a biomarker for aging), mood, and self-esteem. People who take up the challenge presented by diet and exercise prescriptions make huge strides in their physical and emotional recovery; imagine what it does to their independence.

Complementary Therapies

Massage Therapy

Massage therapy increases circulation (blood flow), reduces muscle tension, and helps a person relax. It can be very useful to people who experience problems with rigidity (stiffness). Massage should be part of an overall fitness program that includes regular movement and exercise.

Select a massage therapist who is certified by the American Massage Therapy Association. Talk to the therapist about methods. The care receiver should provide feedback during the massage in the event of any discomfort. Self-massage and massage provided by the caregiver are also possible. Using items such as wooden rollers or hand-held electric massagers will allow you or the person in your care to apply gentle pressure to tight areas of the body. These items can be purchased at most drug or department stores. Massage services are often not covered by health insurance unless they are part of your muscle strengthening prescription recommended by your physical therapist or medical professional.

Tai Chi

Tai chi is a slow, flowing form of ancient Chinese exercise. It aids in flexibility, balance, and relaxation. Several forms of tai chi can be done by anyone regardless of age or physical condition. Classes are often offered at fitness centers, senior centers, and community recreation centers. Speak with the instructor to learn if the type of tai chi he or she teaches is best for the person in your care. Tai chi classes are often available locally. Also visit www.taoist.org to find a class in your area.

Yoga

Yoga is a form of exercise that can be very helpful for persons with chronic illness. It increases flexibility, relaxation, and awareness of breathing and posture. Yoga also can reduce stress. Yoga is self-paced, which means that people can do the poses in their own way and hold the pose for as long as they are comfortable. Yoga can even be done in a chair. It is important to contact the instructor prior to beginning a class. Generally, a beginner class or a class for those with special needs is a good place for your care receiver to start.

> *Tip*
>
> If the person in your care has significant balance impairment, Tai Chi and yoga moves from a chair may be necessary.

Pet Therapy

"Lap" pets, such as dogs and cats, can provide great joy in the lives of their human friends. Having animals in the home improves the mental and emotional health of their owners. It also provides movement and exercise. According to research, pets can

- lower blood pressure and heart rate

- improve mobility and flexibility (through stroking, grooming, and walking the pet)

- satisfy the human need for touch and caring for another

Creative Expression

Creative expression can provide movement and physical activity. Painting on an easel with large, strong strokes stretches the arms and shoulders. "Conducting" the music of a favorite symphony or opera has shown to have a strengthening and aerobic benefit. Singing alone or in a choral group promotes the deep breathing needed for louder speech. Encourage the person in your care to seek creative outlets that fit their talents and abilities.

Exercise and the Daily Routine

A good exercise regimen can help a person maintain mobility.
Some persons may not be able to follow an exercise program due to changes in their physical ability. It may be better for those people to fit exercises and stretching into the daily routine:

- Find a simple activity that the person enjoys, such as walking, gardening, housekeeping, or swimming. As caregiver, you can try to make some of these activities part of the daily routine.

- Sitting and reaching in different directions can stretch the arms and trunk.

- Household chores such as folding laundry, dusting, wiping dishes, or helping with food preparation provide gentle exercise.

- Simple games like balloon volleyball, playing catch with a large, soft ball or blowing soap bubbles are an enjoyable way to get exercise.

- Music creates movement such as marching or dancing. If balance is a problem, try chair dancing. "Conducting" to the beat of up-tempo music provides upper body exercise and good emotional therapy!

- Perform a few extra arm and leg motions during dressing tasks.

A physical therapist can suggest exercises and stretches that will suit the person in your care. Therapists can also provide ways to improve walking and balance, if necessary.

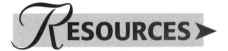

RESOURCES ►

American Dietetic Association
120 South Riverside Plaza, Suite 2000
Chicago, IL 60606-6995
(800) 877-1600
(312) 899-0040
membrshp@eatright.org
www.eatright.org
Call weekdays 8:00 a.m. to 5:00 p.m. CST or fill a online request to locate a registered dietitian in your area.

Area Agency on Aging or the **Cooperative Extension Service**
Your local office offers free counseling by a registered dietitian.

Meals-on-Wheels
413 North Lee Street
Alexandria, VA 22314
(888) 998-6325
(703) 548-5274 (fax)
mowaa@mowaa.org
www.mowaa.org/
Can provide nutritious meals delivered to the home.

The US Department of Agriculture
MyPyramid
www.mypyramid.gov
www.choosemyplate.gov/print-materials-ordering/
mypyramid-archive.html
This replaces the old Food Guide Pyramid. It is a very interactive site to help people make healthy choices consistent with the latest Dietary Guidelines for Americans.

The National Sports Center for the Disabled (NSCD)
Sports Authority Field at Mile High
1801 Mile High Stadium Circle, #1500
Denver, CO 80204
(970) 726-1540
www.nscd.org
info@nscd.org
NSCD is a nonprofit corporation that offers winter and summer recreation. Winter sports include snow skiing, snowshoeing, and cross-country skiing. Summer recreation activities include fishing, hiking, rock climbing, whitewater rafting, camping, mountain biking, sailing, therapeutic horseback riding, and a baseball camp.

The Official Web site of the National Association for Disabled Sailing
http://www.sailing.org/disabled/

Taoist Tai Chi Society of the USA
National Headquarters
2100 Thomasville Road
Tallahassee, Florida 32308-0736
(850) 224-5438 (voice)
(850) 383-1353 (fax)
http://usa.taoist.org/contact.html
Look for local classes; your first class is free. Taoist Tai Chi® incorporates stretching and turning into a sequence of

movements that improve the health of body, mind, and spirit. They reduce tension, improve circulation and balance, and increase strength and flexibility. Over time, these internal arts reach deep inside the body to benefit its entire physiology and restore the calmness and peace of mind often lost through the excessive desires and anxieties of daily life.

The Food Network
http://www.foodnetwork.com/recipes-and-cooking/meat-and-poultry-temperature-guide/index.html
Provides a chart showing temperature options for cooking, using USDA recommendations.

Publications

The Dash Diet
http://dashdiet.org/weight_loss_solution.asp
Billed as one of the best diets for those with high blood pressure, the DASH diet is based on proven research. The diet is designed to speed weight loss and boost metabolism.

A Modification of the Rules of Golf for Golfers with Disabilities
The R&A
St. Andrews
Fife
KY16 9JD
Scotland
www.randa.org Follow the Information for Golfers with Disabilities link under Useful Articles and Tools. This online publication contains permissible modifications to the rules of golf for players with a disability.

Agency for Healthcare Research and
Agency for Healthcare Research and Quality
Office of Communications and Knowledge Transfer

540 Gaither Road, Suite 2000
Rockville, MD 20850.
(301) 427-1104.
http://www.ahrq.gov/index.html

If you don't have access to the Internet, ask your local library or senior center to help you locate a Web site.

Emergencies

Emergencies

*E*mergency situations are common when caring for a person with chronic illness. Many injuries can be avoided through preventive measures (📖 See **Preparing the Home**, p. 113). When a crisis does occur, use common sense, stay calm, and realize that you can help.

> **NOTE** ▶ Make sure 911 is posted on your phone or ideally is on speed-dial. Keep written driving instructions near the phone for how to get to your house. If you have a speakerphone, use the speaker when talking to the dispatcher. This way, you can follow the dispatcher's instructions while attending to the emergency.

When to Call for an Ambulance

Call for an ambulance if a person—

- Becomes unconscious, unarousable
- Has chest pain or pressure
- Has trouble breathing
- Has no signs of breathing (no movement or response to touch or voice)
- Is bleeding severely
- Is vomiting blood or is bleeding from the rectum
- Has fallen and may have broken bones
- Has had a seizure
- Has a severe headache and slurred speech

- Has pressure or severe pain in the abdomen that does not go away

- Has experienced a head injury with altered mental status (lethargy, confusion, combative, unresponsive, headache, vomiting, trouble walking)

OR

- If moving the person could cause further injury

- If traffic or distance would cause a life-threatening delay in getting to the hospital

- If the person is too heavy for you to lift or help

Ambulance service is expensive and may not be covered by insurance. Use it when you believe there is an emergency.

In an emergency:

Step 1: Call 911.
Step 2: Care for the victim.

Also call 911 for emergencies involving fire, explosion, poisonous gas, fallen electrical wires, or other life-threatening situations.

NOTE If the person in your care has signed a Do Not Resuscitate (DNR) order, have it available to show the paramedics. Otherwise, they are required to initiate resuscitation (reviving the person). The order must go with the patient. The Do Not Resuscitate order *must* be with the patient at all times.

In the Emergency Room

Be sure you understand the instructions for care before leaving the emergency room. Call the patient's personal doctor as soon as possible and let him or her know about the emergency room care.

Bring to the emergency room—

- Insurance policy numbers
- A list of medical problems
- A list of medications currently being taken
- The personal physician's name and phone number
- The name and number of a relative or friend of the person in your care

---

We strongly suggest that you take a course in CPR from your local American Red Cross, hospital, or other agency.

Choking (Adult)

- Avoid serving excessive alcohol.
- Make sure the person in your care has a good set of dentures to chew food properly.
- Cut the food into small pieces.
- For a person who has had a stroke, use thickening powder in liquids as directed.
- Do not encourage the person to talk while eating.
- Do not make the person laugh while eating.
- Learn the Heimlich maneuver in CPR class.

Bleeding

If someone is bleeding heavily, protect yourself with rubber gloves, plastic wrap, or layers of cloth. Then—

1. Apply direct pressure over the wound with a clean cloth.

2. Apply another clean cloth on top of the blood-soaked cloth, keeping the pressure firm.

3. If no bones are broken, elevate (raise) the injured limb to decrease blood flow.

4. Call 911 for an ambulance.

5. Apply a bandage snugly over the dressing.

6. Wash your hands with soap and water as soon as possible after providing care.

7. Avoid contact with blood-soaked objects.

8. Mouth bleeding – when able apply pressure to area bleeding in mouth

9. Mouth injuries have a potential for broken, loose or knocked out teeth. Be aware of potential to choke.

10. Check mouth for missing teeth.

11. Rinse mouth with water or saline.

12. Loose tooth, ask person to bite down on gauze pad. Contact a dentist.

13. Missing tooth, apply pressure at empty socket with gauze.

14. Place tooth in water or milk and get person to an Emergency Department or dentist.

Shock

Shock may be associated with heavy bleeding, hives, shortness of breath, dizziness, swelling, thirst, and chest pain. The signs of shock are:

- Restlessness and irritability

- Confusion, altered consciousness

- Pale, cool, moist skin

- Rapid breathing and weakness

If these signs are present—

1. Have the person lie down.

2. Control any bleeding.

3. Keep the person warm.

4. Elevate the legs about 12 to 14 inches unless the neck or back has been injured.

5. Do not give the person anything to eat or drink.

6. Call 911.

Burns/Skin/Eyes

1. Stop the burning process by pouring large amounts of cold water over the burn.

2. Do *not* remove clothing stuck to the burned area.

3. Cover the burn with a dry, clean covering.

4. Keep the person warm.

5. For **chemical burns to the eyes,** flush the eyes with large amounts of cool running water from the faucet or shower.

OR

Immerse the person's face in water and have the person open and close his eyes.

6. Call 911 for transport to hospital.

Chest Pain

Any chest pain that lasts more than a few minutes is related to the heart until proven otherwise. CALL 911 IMMEDIATELY. Don't wait to see if it goes away. Danger signs include—

- Pain radiating from the chest down the arms, up the neck to the jaw, and into the back

- Crushing, squeezing chest pain or heavy pressure in the chest

- Shortness of breath, sweating, nausea and vomiting, weakness

- Bluish, pale skin

- Skin that is moist

- Excessive perspiration

If the person is unresponsive (no movement or response to touch or voice, no pulse), **call 911** and be prepared to start CPR. If *untrained* in CPR, then provide Hands-Only™ CPR—uninterrupted chest compressions, hard and fast, about 100 a minute, until rescue personnel arrive. If CPR *trained*, give 30 chest compressions, hard and fast, at least 100 times per minute, followed by 2 Rescue Breaths.Repeat compressions and ventilation (30:2) until help arrives or the person responds.

To view the **American Heart Association's** Hands-Only™ CPR video, visit www.heart.org and search Hands-Only.

Falls and Related Injuries

Preventive measures include—

- Staying in when it is rainy or icy outside

- Having regular vision screening check-ups for eyeglasses

- Using separate reading glasses and other regular glasses if bifocals make it difficult to see the floor

- Being cautious when walking on wet floors

- Wearing good foot support when walking

- Being aware that new shoes are slippery and crepe-soled shoes can cause the toe to catch

- Having foot pain problems corrected

- Keeping toenails trimmed and feet healthy for good balance

A good way to tell if a part of the body has been injured in a fall is to compare it with an uninjured part. For example, compare the injured leg with the uninjured leg. Do they look and feel the same? Do they move the same way?

When you suspect a *broken bone*, follow these steps:

- If the person *cannot* move or use the injured limb, keep it from moving. Do not straighten a deformed arm or leg. Splint an injury in the position you find it.

- Support the injured part above and below the site of the injury by using folded towels, blankets or pillows

- If the person is face down, roll him over with the "log rolling" technique (see illustration). If you have no one to help you and the victim is breathing adequately, leave the person in the same position.

- If the person does not complain of neck pain but is feeling sick to the stomach, turn the person on one side.

- If the person complains of neck pain, keep his neck steady by putting a few pillows on either side of his head. Keep the head flat.

- Place a piece of cloth on the injury site and apply ice over the cloth.

- Keep the person warm with a blanket and make the person as comfortable as possible.

- Make a splint with cardboard or rolled-up newspaper.

▶ *Log rolling technique—Turning a person safely from the stomach onto the back.*

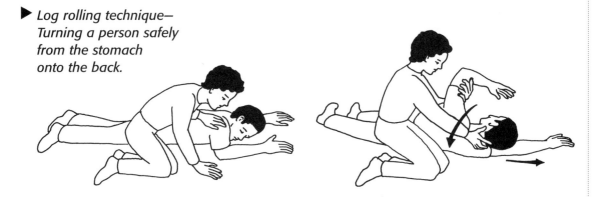

NOTE If an arm or shoulder is splinted, you might consider transporting the person by car. For neck, hip, thigh, back, and pelvic injuries, use an ambulance because the person needs to lie flat.

Fainting

Fainting can be caused by—

- A heart attack

- Medications

- Low blood sugar

- Standing up quickly

- Straining to have a bowel movement

- Dehydration

To some extent, fainting can be prevented.

- Ask the doctor if medications that do not cause fainting can be prescribed.

- Monitor blood sugar levels.

- Avoid constipation.

- Do not let the person stand up or sit up too rapidly.

If a fainting spell occurs:

1. Do not try to place the person in a sitting position. Instead, immediately lay him down flat.

2. Check the person's airway, breathing, and pulse.

3. Turn the person on his side.

4. Elevate the legs.

5. Cover him with a blanket if the room or floor is cold.

6. Do not give fluids.

7. **Call 911** if person is having difficulty breathing, not breathing, or not responding to your voice and touch.

8. If the person is unresponsive (no movement or response to touch or voice, no pulse), **call 911** and be prepared to start CPR. If *untrained* in CPR, then provide Hands-Only™ CPR—uninterrupted chest compressions, hard and fast, about 100 a minute, until rescue personnel arrive. If CPR *trained*, give 30 chest compressions, hard and fast, at least 100 times per minute, followed by 2 Rescue Breaths.Repeat compressions and ventilation (30:2) until help arrives or the person responds.

Hypothermia

Hypothermia occurs when a person's body temperature falls below normal (around 98.6°F). Conditions that may alter the person's body response to cold are:

- Hypothyroidism (low thyroid activity)
- Arthritis
- Dizziness and resulting falls
- Excessive alcohol
- Stroke
- Head injuries
- Medications that cause poor body-temperature regulation

To prevent hypothermia—

- Keep the house temperature no lower than 65°F (70°F if the person is ill).
- Have him wear warm clothes, and place wool leg warmers on his arms and legs for extra warmth.
- Use warm blankets when the person is in bed.
- Have him wear a warm hat outside or a knit hat indoors to keep from losing body heat.
- Provide a balanced diet.
- Provide exercise of some sort.

Signs of hypothermia include impaired judgment, shivering, cold pale skin, slow breathing and pulse, weakness, drowsiness, and confusion. If these signs are present, do the following:

1. Wrap the person in blankets, notify the doctor, give warm fluids, and increase room temperature.

2. Avoid rubbing the person's skin.

3. Do not rewarm the person rapidly. Use a heater on low or warm hot-water bottles on the chest and abdomen. Warm slowly and handle the person carefully.

4. Do not give the person alcohol.

5. Be alert to signs of a heart attack (📖 See p. 323).

Heat Stroke

Some medications can increase the likelihood of heat stroke. To prevent heat stroke—

- Ask the doctor if the medicine the person is taking can increase the risk of heat stroke.

- Use clothing made of breathable lightweight fabrics.

- Use a fan, damp compresses, or an air conditioner.

- Have the person drink 6–8 glasses of water even if not feeling thirsty.

- Avoid alcohol, caffeine, and smoking because they speed dehydration.

- Avoid activity during the hottest part of the day.

Signs of heat stroke include headache, nausea, and sudden dizziness. Consult the doctor immediately to determine whether it is a serious condition. Call 911 if you suspect heat stroke.

Oral Injuries/Teeth

A person with a mouth injury may have knocked-out teeth, broken or loose teeth. This can be a choking hazard.

If you suspect an oral injury, immediately take these steps:

1. Put on gloves.

2. Check the mouth for loose teeth, broken teeth or any missing teeth.

3. Rinse the mouth with clean water or saline.

4. If tooth is loose, have the person bite down on a piece of gauze to keep the tooth in place and call the dentist.

5. If tooth is chipped, clean the injured area and call a dentist.

6. If a tooth is missing, apply gauze with pressure to stop the bleeding from the empty tooth socket.

7. If tooth has come out, place the tooth in clean water or cup of milk and immediately take the person and tooth to a dentist.

8. Whenever you handle the tooth, it is important to hold the top part or the tooth (the crown) and avoid touching the root of the tooth which may have ligaments on the tooth that will help reattach the tooth.

Poisons

If you suspect poisoning, immediately take these steps:

1. Determine **what** was swallowed, **how much,** and at **what time**.

2. Check the person's airway. (Are there signs of breathing, coughing, moving?)

3. Contact the nearest Poison Control Center or call 911 for treatment; have the container of the suspected poison at hand.

4. Follow up with the doctor.

5. If the person is unresponsive (no movement or response to touch or voice, no pulse), **call 911** and be prepared to start CPR. If *untrained* in CPR, then provide Hands-Only™ CPR—uninterrupted chest compressions, hard and fast, about 100 a minute, until rescue personnel arrive. If CPR *trained*, give 30 chest compressions, hard and fast, at least 100 times per minute, followed by 2 Rescue Breaths.Repeat compressions and ventilation (30:2) until help arrives or the person responds.

Seizures

A seizure usually lasts from 1 to 5 minutes. If it lasts longer than you are comfortable with or more than 7 minutes, call 911 for an ambulance.

1. Remove all objects that might cause the person to injure himself.

2. Place pillows and blankets around him to protect him.

3. Do **not** hold or restrain the person.

4. Do **not** place anything in the person's mouth.

5. Always check for **breathing** and **signs of circulation** after the seizure stops.

6. Reassure and comfort the person.

7. If the person is unresponsive (no movement or response to touch or voice, no pulse), **call 911** and be prepared to start CPR. If *untrained* in CPR, then provide Hands-Only™ CPR—uninterrupted chest compressions, hard and fast, about 100 a minute, until rescue personnel arrive. If CPR *trained*, give 30 chest compressions, hard and fast, at least 100 times per minute, followed by 2 Rescue Breaths.Repeat compressions and ventilation (30:2) until help arrives or the person responds.

Stroke

Strokes occur when the blood flow to the brain is interrupted by a clogged or burst blood vessel. Strokes cannot always be prevented, but the chances of their occurring can be lessened through—

- A balanced diet
- Avoidance of stress
- Periodic checkups
- Regular exercise
- Regular use of a prescribed blood pressure medicine

Suspect a stroke when the person in your care—

- Has a sudden and severe headache
- Does not respond to simple statements
- Has a seizure
- Is suddenly incontinent (unable to control bladder and bowel)
- Has paralysis in (cannot move) an arm or leg
- Cannot grip equally with both hands
- Appears droopy on one side of the face
- Has slurred speech or blurred vision
- Is confused
- Has an unsteady gait
- Has trouble swallowing
- Has loss of balance or coordination when combined with one of the other signs

The chance of recovery from a stroke is greatly increased if the person has immediate help.

1. Keep the person in the position you found him in.

2. Reassure him and keep him calm.

3. If he has trouble breathing, open his airway, tilt his head, and lift his chin.

4. Call 911. Get the person to medical care as soon as possible.

5. If the person is unresponsive (no movement or response to touch or voice, no pulse), **call 911** and be prepared to start CPR. If *untrained* in CPR, then provide Hands-Only™ CPR—uninterrupted chest compressions, hard and fast, about 100 a minute, until rescue personnel arrive. If CPR *trained*, give 30 chest compressions, hard and fast, at least 100 times per minute, followed by 2 Rescue Breaths.Repeat compressions and ventilation (30:2) until help arrives or the person responds.

6. If breathing resumes, place the person on one side to prevent choking. This also helps keep the tongue out of the airway.

Checklist **Home First Aid Kit**

Buy or make a home first-aid kit. Note on the box the date when the item was purchased. Check and replenish your supplies at least once a year. These should include the following:

✔ Adhesive tape

✔ Antibiotic ointment

✔ Antiseptic wipes or towelettees

✔ Bandage, compression (2-, 3-, and 4-inch)

✔ Band-Aids®

✔ Benadryl (Diphenhydrmine)

✔ Cotton balls and cotton-tipped swabs

✔ Disinfectant for cleaning wounds

✔ Disposable gloves

✔ Emergency telephone numbers

✔ Eye pads

✔ Gloves, disposable—Instant ice packs

✔ List of current medications

✔ Petroleum jelly or other lubricant

✔ Pocket mask/face mask

✔ Rolled gauze and elastic bandages

✔ Safety pins in assorted sizes

✔ Scissors

✔ oap or hand sanitizer

✔ Sterile gauze bandages (nonstick, 4 × 4-inch)

✔ Syrup of ipecac

✔ Saline nose drops

✔ Tape

✔ Thermometer

✔ Tongue depressors

✔ 3-ounce rubber bulb to rinse out wounds

✔ Triangular bandage

✔ Tweezers and needle

Body Mechanics—Positioning, Moving, and Transfers

Body Mechanics—Positioning, Moving, and Transfers

Body Mechanics for the Caregiver

Body mechanics involves standing and moving one's body so as to prevent injury, avoid fatigue, and make the best use of strength. When you learn how to control and balance your own body, you can safely control and move another person. Back injuries to nursing home aides are common, so when doing any lifting be sure to use proper body mechanics.

General Rules

- Never lift more than you can comfortably handle.

- Create a base of support by standing with your feet 8–12 inches (shoulder width) apart with one foot a half step ahead of the other.

Proper foot position ▶

- DO NOT let your back do the heavy work—USE YOUR LEGS. (The back muscles are not your strongest muscles.)

- If the bed is low, put one foot on a footstool. This relieves pressure on your lower back.

- Consider using a support belt for your back.

Helpful Caregiver Advice for Moving a Person

These pointers are for the *caregiver* only. Be sure to see the following pages for the steps for a specific

◀ **1**
- Tell the person what you are going to do.
- Before starting a move, count with the person, "1-2-3."

◀ **2**
- To feel in control, get close to the person you are lifting.
- While lifting, keep your back in a neutral position (arched normally, not stiff), knees bent, weight balanced on both feet. Tighten your stomach and back muscles to maintain a correct support position.
- Use your arms to support the person.
- Again, *let your legs do the lifting*.

◀ **3**
- Pivot (turn on one foot) instead of twisting your body.
- Breathe deeply.
- Keep your shoulders relaxed.
- When a lot of assistance is needed with transfers, tie a strong belt or a transfer belt around the person's waist and hold it as you complete the transfer.

Prevention of Back and Neck Injuries

To prevent injuries to yourself, get plenty of rest and maintain:

- Good nutrition

- Physical fitness

- Good body mechanics

- A program for managing stress

Common Treatments for Caregiver Back Pain

If you **do** experience back pain:

- Apply a cold ice pack to the injured area for 10 minutes every hour (you can use a bag of frozen vegetables).

- Get short rest periods in a comfortable position.

- Stand with your feet about shoulder width apart and hands on hips, bend backwards. Do 3–5 repetitions several times a day.

- Take short, frequent walks on a level surface.

- Avoid sitting for long periods because sitting is one of the worst healing positions.

As the caregiver, you should seek training from a physical therapist to provide this type of care to reduce the risk of injury to yourself or the person in your care. The therapist will correct any mistakes you make and can take into account special problems. To determine the best procedure for you to use, the therapist will consider the physical condition of the person you care for and the furniture and room arrangements in the home.

Moving a Person

When you have to move someone—either in bed or out of bed—remember these tips:

- Plan the move and know what you can and cannot do.

- Let the person do as much work as he is capable of.

- Avoid letting the person put his arms around your neck or grab you.

- Use a transfer belt to balance and support the person.

- Place transfer surfaces (wheelchair and bed) close together.

- Check wheelchair position, **brakes locked**, armrests and footrests swung out of the way.

- Let the person look to the place where he is being transferred.

- If the person is able, place his hands on the bed or chair so he can assist in the movement. If the person has had a stroke or is afraid, have him clasp his hands close to his chest.

- Ask the person to *push* rather than *pull* on the bed rails, the chair, or you.

- Work at the person's level and speed and check for pain.

- Avoid sudden jerking motions.

- Never pull on the person's arms or shoulders.

- Correctly position the person. (This helps the body regain lost function and helps prevent additional function loss.)

- Have the person wear shoes with good treads or sturdy slippers.

NOTE To encourage independence, let the person assist as she is able. It's okay for the person to stand up partly and sit back down.

Positioning a Person in Bed

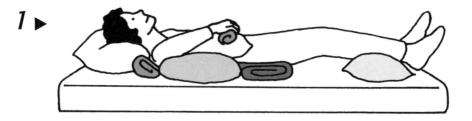

1 ▶

- Place a small pillow under the person's head, keeping his spine neutral.

- Place a small pillow lengthwise under the calf of the weak leg, let the heel hang off the end of the pillow to prevent pressure, and loosen the top sheet to avoid pressure on the toes.

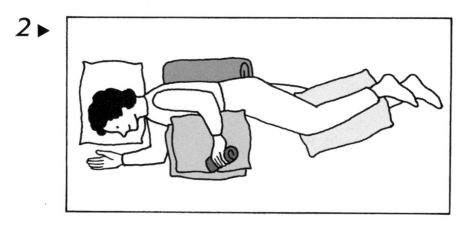

2 ▶

- Fold a bath towel under the hip of the person's weak side.

- Place the weak arm and elbow on a pillow higher than the heart.

Positioning a Person on His or Her Strong Side

1. Place a small pillow under the person's head.

2. Keep the person's head in alignment with the spine.

3. Place a rolled pillow at the back to prevent rolling.

4. Place a pillow in front to keep the arm the same height as the shoulder joint.

5. Place a medium pillow lengthwise between the knees, legs, and ankles. (The person's knees may be bent slightly.)

Positioning a Person on His or Her Weak Side

1. Use the same positioning as described above.

2. Change the person's position frequently because he may not be aware of pressure, pain, or skin irritation.

Moving a person in bed can injure the person in care or the caregiver if certain basic rules are not followed:

- Never grab or pull the person's arm or leg.

- If the medical condition allows, raise the foot of the bed slightly to prevent the person from sliding down.

- If moving him is difficult, get him out of bed and back in the wheelchair and start over by putting him in bed closer to the headboard.

Moving a Person Up in Bed

1. Tell the person what you are going to do.

2. Lower the head of the bed to a flat position and remove the pillow—never try to move the person "uphill."

3. If possible, raise the bed and **lock the wheels**.

4. Tell the person to bend his knees and brace his feet firmly against the mattress to help push.

5. Stand at the side of the bed and place one hand behind the person's back and the other underneath the buttocks.

6. Bend your knees and keep your back in a neutral position.

7. Count "1-2-3" and have the person push with his feet and pull with his hands toward the head of the bed.

8. Replace the pillow under his head.

Using Two People to Move an Unconscious Person

1
- Tell the person what you are going to do even if the person seems to be unconscious.

- Remove the pillow.

- If possible, raise the bed and **lock the wheels**.

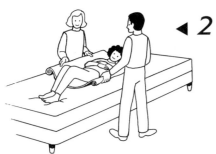

◀ *2*
- Stand on either side of the bed.

- Face the head of the bed, with feet 8–12 inches apart, knees bent, back in a neutral position.

- Roll the sides of the draw sheet up to the person's body.

◀ *3*
- Grab the draw sheet with your palms up.

- Count "1-2-3" and then shift your body weight from the back to the front leg, keeping your arms and back in a locked position. Together, slide the person smoothly up the bed.

- Replace pillows under the person's head.

- Position the person comfortably.

> **NOTE** A drawsheet—a sheet folded several times and positioned under the person to be moved in bed—prevents irritation to his skin. The sheet should be positioned from the shoulders to just below the knees.

Moving an Unconscious Person Alone

1. If possible, raise the whole bed and **lock the wheels**.

2. Remove the pillow.

3. Face the front of the bed, with feet 8–12 inches apart, knees bent, back in a neutral position.

4. Roll the edge of the draw sheet and grab it.

5. Slide your arms under the draw sheet and the person's shoulders and back.

6. Count "1-2-3" and then shift your body weight from your back to front leg, keeping your arms and back in a locked position.

7. Slide the person to the top of the bed.

8. Replace the pillow.

9. Position the person comfortably.

PREVENTING BACK INJURIES
Having the person grab a trapeze to help with the move is easiest and safest for your back. (📖 See p. 139)

Moving the Person to One Side of the Bed on His or Her Back

1 • Place your feet 8–12 inches apart, knees bent, back in a neutral position.

• Slide your arms under the person's back to her far shoulder blade. (Bend your knees and hips to lower yourself to the person's level.)

• Slide the person's shoulders toward you by rocking your weight to your back foot.

2 • Use the same procedure at the person's buttocks and feet.

• Always keep your knees bent and your back in a neutral position.

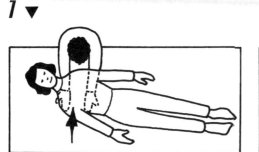

1 ▼   **2** ▼

Moving the person

Rolling Technique

1. Move the person to one side of the bed as in the above procedure.

2. Bend the person's knees.

3. Hold the person at her hip and shoulder blade on the far side of the body.

4. Roll the person *toward* you to make sure she does not fall off the bed.

Raising the Person's Head and Shoulders

1. If possible, ask the person to lift her head and dig both elbows into the bed to support her body.

2. Face the head of the bed, feet 8–12 inches apart, knees bent, back in neutral.

3. Help the person lift her shoulders by placing your hands and forearms under the pillow and her shoulder blades.

4. Use bent knees, back in neutral, and locked arms to assist the lift.

5. Adjust the pillow.

Helping a Person Sit Up

1. Tell the person what you are going to do.

2. Bend the person's knees.

3. Roll her on her side so she is facing you.

4. Reach one arm under her shoulder blade.

5. Place the other arm in back of her knees.

6. Position your feet 8–12 inches apart with your center of gravity close to the bed and the person.

7. Keep your back in a neutral position.

8. Count "1-2-3" and shift your weight to your back leg.

9. Shift the person's legs over the edge of the bed while pulling her shoulders to a sitting position.

10. Remain in front of her until she is stabilized.

Getting Adequate Rest

It is common for the elderly or a person with a disability to have trouble turning over or getting in and out of bed. These tips may help:

- If the person is having trouble getting in and out of bed or turning over in bed, talk to the health care provider. Medication may have to be adjusted.

- A satin sheet or piece of satin material tucked across the middle of the bed can make it easier for the person to turn over.

- Flannel sheets and heavy blankets can make it more difficult to turn over.

- Make sure the path from the bed to the bathroom is well lighted. Use a nightlight or leave open a closet door with the light left on.

- Keep the bedroom floor clear of things that could cause a person to trip or fall. Don't leave shoes, books, or magazines on the floor.

Getting Up from Bed and Lying Down

To help the person in your care get up from bed, explain and repeat the following steps:

1. Bend knees up. Place feet flat on bed.

2. Turn on to side. Reach arm across body to assist rolling.

3. Move feet off edge of bed.

4. Use arms to push self into sitting position. (A half-side rail or chair fastened to the side of the bed may help.)

To help the person lie down in bed, explain and repeat the following steps:

1. Sit on edge of bed.

2. Lift legs into bed (one at a time may be easier).

3. Lie down with head on pillow.

4. Slide legs into center of bed (moving one leg at a time may be easier.)

Helping Someone Get Into Bed

1. Have the person approach the bed as if he were going to sit in a chair. He should feel the mattress behind both legs.

2. Have the person slowly lower himself to a seated position on the bed, using his arms to control the lowering.

3. Tell him to lean on his forearm while allowing his trunk to lean down to the side.

4. As the trunk goes down, the legs will want to go up, like a seesaw.

5. Do not have the person place his knees up on the mattress first. In other words, he shouldn't "crawl" into bed.

Helping Someone Get Out of Bed

1. Have the person bend the knees up, feet flat on the bed.

2. Tell him to roll onto his side toward the edge of the bed by letting his knees fall to that side. Tell him to turn his head and look in the direction he is rolling.

3. Have him lower his feet from the bed and push with his arms into a sitting position.

4. A straight-back chair anchored at the side of the bed or a bed rail can help the person roll more easily.

Transfers

Transferring a person in and out of bed is an important care-giver activity. It can be done fairly easily if these instructions are followed. Use the same procedure for all transfers so that a routine is set up.

Transfers Using a Mechanical Lift

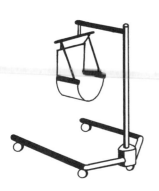

1. Tell the person what you are going to do.

2. Place the chair next to the bed with the back of the chair in line with the headboard of the bed. **Lock the wheels.**

3. Place a blanket or sheet over the chair.

4. Turn the person on one side toward the edge of the bed.

5. Fan-fold a sling and place it at the person's back.

6. Roll her to her other side, pull the sling out flat, and center it under her body.

7. Attach the sling to the mechanical lift with the hooks in place and facing out through the metal frame.

8. Fold the person's arms across her chest.

9. Using the crank, lift her out of bed.

10. Guide the legs. Lower her onto the chair.

11. Remove the hooks from the frame of the mechanical lift.

12. Leave the person in the chair with the sling under her, comfortably adjusted.

13. To get the person back in the bed, put the hooks facing out through the metal frame of the sling.

14. Raise the person using the crank.

15. Guide her legs. Lower her onto the bed.

16. Remove the hooks from the frame.

17. Remove the sling from under the person by turning her from side to side on the bed.

18. Properly position her with pillows. (📖 See p. 340)

For lift instructions see the *Positioning and Transfer Guide* that comes with your mechanical lift.

Helping a Person Stand

Help only as much as needed but guard the person from falling.

1. Have her sit on the edge of the chair or bed. Let her rest a moment if she feels lightheaded.

2. Instruct her to push off with her hands from the bed or chair armrests.

3. Position your knee between her knees.

4. Face her and support the weak knee against one or both of your knees as needed.

5. Put your arms around the person's waist or use a transfer belt.

6. Keep your back in a neutral position.

7. At the count of "1-2-3," instruct the person to stand up while pulling her toward you and pushing your knees into her knee if needed.

 NOTE If during a transfer you start to "lose" the person, do not try to hold her up. Instead, lower her to the floor.

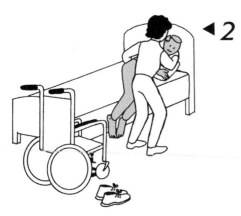

8. Once she is upright, have her keep her knee locked straight.

9. Support and balance her as needed.

Helping a Person Sit

1. Reverse the process described in Helping a Person Stand.

2. Direct the person to feel for the chair or bed with the back of the legs.

3. Direct the person to reach back with both hands to the bed or chair armrests and slowly sit.

Transferring from Bed to Wheelchair with a Transfer Belt

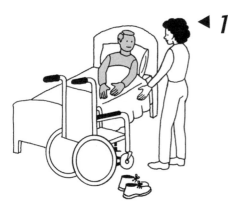

◀ 1
- Place the wheelchair at a 45-degree angle to the bed so that the person will be transferring to his stronger side.

- **Lock the wheels** of the chair and the bed.

- Tell the person what you are going to do.

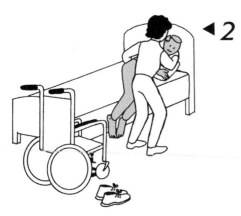

◀ 2
- Put on his shoes while he is still lying down if he is weak or unstable.

- Bring him to a sitting position with his legs over the edge of the bed.

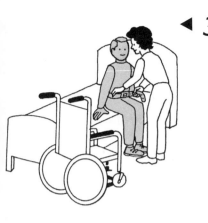

◀ **3** • Let him rest a moment if he feels lightheaded.

• Use a **transfer belt** for a person needing a lot of support.

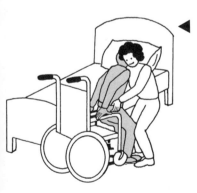

◀ **4** • Bring him to a standing position as described on page 349.

◀ **5** • Have him reach for the chair arm and pivot. A very fast pivot may frighten the person, or cause you to lose knee control and fall with a person who is totally dependent.

• Support him with your arms and knees as needed.

• Adjust him comfortably in the chair.

NOTE ▶ If the person starts to slide off the edge of the bed before or after the transfer, lay his upper torso across the bed to prevent him from falling to the floor.

Transferring from Wheelchair to Bed

1. Reverse the process described in Transfer from Bed to Wheelchair.

2. Place the chair at a 45-degree angle to the bed so the person is on his stronger side. **Lock the wheels**.

3. Get into a position to provide a good base of support; use good body mechanics.

4. Have the person stand, reach for the bed, and pivot.

5. Support and guide him as needed.

6. Adjust the person in bed with pillows.

Transferring from Bed to Wheelchair Without a Transfer Belt

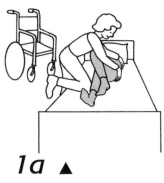

- Place the wheelchair at a 45-degree angle to the bed so that the person will be transferring to his stronger side.

- **Lock the wheels** of the chair (you can use a wheel block) and the wheels of the bed.

- Tell the person what you are going to do.

- Bring him to a sitting position with his legs over the edge of the bed following steps a, b, c, and d.

1a ▲

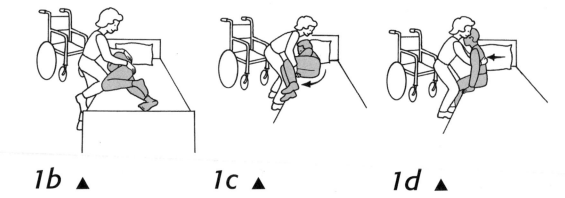

1b ▲   **1c** ▲   **1d** ▲

- Let him rest a moment if he feels lightheaded.

- Put his shoes on.

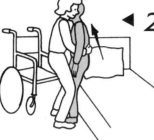

◀ **2**
- Put your arms around his chest and clasp your hands behind his back.

- Support the leg that is farther from the wheelchair between your legs.

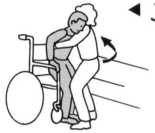

◀ **3**
- Lean back, shift your leg, and lift.
- Pivot toward the chair.

◀ **4**
- Bend your knees and let him bend toward you.

- Lower the person into the wheelchair.

- Adjust him comfortably in the chair.

NOTE ▷ As the person becomes stronger, you can provide less assistance. However, use the same body positioning to support the person's weaker side.

Transferring from Wheelchair to Bed with a Transfer Board

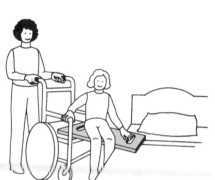

1. As much as possible, make the bed and the chair the same height.

2. Place the wheelchair at a 45° angle to the bed so that the person will be transferring to her stronger side.

3. **Lock the wheels** of the chair (you can use a wheel block) and the wheels of the bed.

4. Tell the person what you are going to do.

5. Remove the armrest nearest the bed.

6. Remove her feet from the footrests and swing the footrests out of the way.

7. Have the person lift her hip and place the board under the hip with the other end of the board on the bed.

8. MAKE SURE SHE DOESN'T PUT HER FINGERS UNDER THE BOARD.

9. Ask her to put her hands on the board with the hands close to her sides.

10. Ask her to lean slightly forward and to make a series of small pushes off the board by straightening her elbows and inching along the board toward the bed.

11. When she is on the bed, ask her to lean over onto her elbow and pull the transfer board out from under her bottom.

12. Adjust her comfortably in the bed.

Transferring from a Wheelchair to a Car

Be sure the car is parked on a level surface without cracks or potholes.

1
- Open the passenger door as far as possible.

- Move the left side of the wheelchair as close to the car seat as possible.

- **Lock the chair's wheels.**

- Move both footrests out of the way.

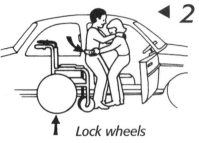

Lock wheels

2
- Position yourself facing the person.

- Tell him what you are going to do.

- Bending your knees and hips, lower yourself to his level.

- By grasping the transfer belt around his waist help him stand while straightening your hips and knees.

- If his legs are weak, brace his knees with your knees.

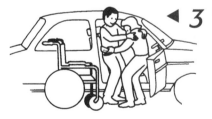

3
- While he is standing, turn him so he can be eased down to sit on the car seat. GUIDE HIS HEAD so it is not bumped.

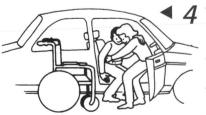

4
- Lift his legs into the car by putting your hands under his knees.

- Move him to face the front.

- Put on his seat belt.

- Close door carefully.

355

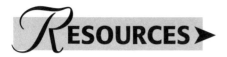

RESOURCES ➤

American Academy of Orthopedic Surgeons
6300 N. River Road
Rosemont, IL 60018
(800) 346-AAOS (800-346-2267)
(847) 823-7186
(847) 823-8125 (fax)
www.aaos.org
Offers a free booklet, "Lift It Safe," on lifting procedures for home-based caregivers.

Mayo Clinic (Burns)
http://www.mayoclinic.com

American Physical Therapy Association
www.apta.org
http://www.moveforwardpt.com/Default.aspx
The Web site provides a handy "Ask a PT?" link.

If you don't have access to the Internet, ask your local library or senior center to help you locate a Web site.

Hospice and Palliative Care

Hospice and Palliative Care

Preparing for Hospice Care

Although terminal illness is a difficult thing to cope with, it also gives the person who is terminally ill and the family time to examine life, establish priorities, and renew or strengthen relationships. During this time, you can help in easing the transition by participating in choices in hospice care. A hospice team can help ensure that the person in your care is as comfortable as possible during this period. It can also guide the patient and family's choices for final arrangements.

When an Illness Takes a Turn for the Worse

When a serious illness becomes life threatening, a person will go through many physical, emotional, and spiritual changes. Decisions to end medical treatment, seek hospice care, or to withdraw life support may need to be made. It's best to talk over these decisions with the physicians and family of the person in your care well before there is a health care crisis.

Discussing the Person's Wishes

- When possible, discuss the person's and the family's wishes before an illness reaches the final phase.

- Does the person have a health care proxy?

- Is there a living will or medical power of attorney?

- What would the person's choices be regarding life support?

- Would the person want to stay at home or enter a facility?

The Principles of Hospice Care

Hospice has always recognized the importance of including the ill person, the family, and other loved ones in the care plan. Caregiving for someone who is dying can be demanding and it's important for everyone involved with a terminal illness to take proper care of his needs.

Hospice services can provide expert, compassionate care and make it possible for a dying person to remain at home. The earlier hospice care begins, the more it can help in providing the care needed at this time. It can also help loved ones enjoy the best quality of life as a family unit.

Questions to Ask When Choosing a Program

In 2011, the number of hospice programs nationwide continued to grow—from the first program in 1974 to over 5,300. The hospice program in your community can provide information and help you answer some of the difficult decisions that accompany terminal illness and dying. Here are some questions you can ask in selecting hospice care:

- Is the agency licensed and accredited by a nationally recognized organization?

- Are they Medicare certified?

- What are their billing policies and payment plans?

- Can they provide references, such as local hospital and care centers, institutions, and caregivers?

- How do they decide whether an individual is ready for hospice care?

- How are their caregivers supervised?

- What are their expectations about the family's sharing in caregiving?

- Are you comfortable with the program? Does it feel like the right fit?

What Hospice Care Provides

Hospice is a concept of medical care that delivers comfort and support to people in the final stages of a terminal illness—and to their families. Care is delivered by a team of specially trained medical professionals who focus on easing pain and managing symptoms. They provide medical, emotional, psychological, and spiritual care to the person and family. They assist the family in coping with their coming loss and their grief afterward.

Most hospice care is provided in the home, but hospice care can also be provided in nursing homes, hospitals, home care agencies, and hospice facilities. The person who is ill and the family are the core of the hospice team and are at the center of all decision making.

Although a family member or other caregiver cares for the person on a daily basis, a hospice nurse is available 24 hours a day to provide advice and make visits. Hospice services include

- Physician services

- Nursing services

- Medical social services

- Home health aide and homemaker services

- Spiritual, dietary, and other counseling

- Physical, occupational, and speech–language therapy

- Medicine for controlling pain

- Medical supplies and appliances

- Ongoing care at home during periods of crisis

- Special services for grief counseling

- Trained volunteers for companionship, errands, or respite

- Short-term inpatient care

- Bereavement (grief) services for the family (or loved ones) for up to a year after death

Although the attending physician typically refers a person to hospice, a family member, friend, or caregiver may also make the referral to hospice. The hospice nurse will contact the doctor for an order for care if that is the wish of the terminally ill person. Any terminal disease or illness qualifies.

Criteria for Admission to a Hospice Care Program

To qualify for hospice care, this condition must be met:

The person must be certified as terminally ill by his or her doctor and the hospice medical director. "Terminally ill" means having a life expectancy of 6 months or less if the disease runs its normal course.

Hospice care involves palliative care (pain and symptom relief). To qualify for Medicare, your physician must recertify you at the beginning of each benefit period (two periods of 90 days, followed by one of 30 days, and an indefinite fourth period). A patient may leave hospice care if his or her condition improves, then reenter if the condition worsens.

Your disease does not need to be terminal for you to qualify for palliative care and, in the United States, some palliative treatments are covered by Medicare. In some cases, palliative treatments can be used to alleviate the side effects of curative treatment, such as relieving the nausea associated with chemotherapy, which may help you tolerate more aggressive or longer-term treatment.

How to Pay for Hospice Care

Hospice care is a benefit under Medicare to beneficiaries with a very limited life expectancy. To receive Medicare payments, the agency or organization must be approved by Medicare to provide hospice services. Under Medicare, hospice is primarily a program of care delivered in the person's home with only short stays in the hospital by a Medicare-approved hospice to provide comfort and relief from pain.

The out-of-pocket expense for the patient may be a co-payment for patient respite care and prescription drugs. At this time, there are no deductibles under the Medicare hospice program. Hospice services can be provided without charge if you have limited or nonexistent financial resources. If you are unable to pay, most hospices will provide for you using funds raised from community donations and charitable foundations.

When All Requirements Are Met, Medicare Covers:

- Doctor services

- Nursing care

- Medical supplies and equipment

- Drugs for symptom management and pain relief (palliative)

- Home health aide and homemaker services

- Physical and occupational therapy

- Speech–language pathology services

- Social worker service

- Dietary and counseling services

- Psychological counseling for emotional support to patient and family

- Spiritual counseling to patient and family

- Respite services for the family

- Volunteer assistance for companionship and respite

The physician must recertify the person's terminal condition. Hospice is also covered under Medicaid in 41 states and by most insurance plans and HMOs.

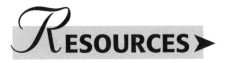

$\mathscr{R}$ESOURCES >

American Cancer Society
(800) 227-2345
www.cancer.org

The University of Texas MD Anderson Center
1515 Holcombe Boulevard
Houston, TX 77030
(877) 632-6789
(713) 792-2121
www.mdanderson.org

Hospice Foundation of America
1710 Rhode Island Ave., NW
Washington, DC 20036
(800) 854-3402
(202) 457-5811
hfaoffice@hospicefoundation.org
www.hospicefoundation.org
Provides information and referral service, resources on end-of-life care, a search engine to end-of-life Web sites, and free brochures on hospice, volunteering, and bereavement.

The National Cancer Institute
Cancer Information Service
(800) 4-CANCER (422-6237)
www.cancernet.gov

Provides free publications and information about cancer and cancer-related resources. Inquiries are handled by trained information specialists. LiveHelp Online Chat and Spanish-speaking staff are available.

National Hospice and Palliative Care Organization
1731 King Street
Alexandria, VA 22314
(800) 658-8898 (hotline)
703-827-1500
www.nhpco.org

Solutions Center
(800) 646-6460
(703) 837-1233 (fax)
Nhpco_info@nhpco.org
www.nhpco.org
Provides information on hospice, referrals to local hospices, and outreach hospice services to families of the dying.

The Help Guide (Resources from A-Z)
http://www.helpguide.org/
A Web site that has grown from a small local project to an internationally recognized resource serving over 50 million people a year.

Call your local **Social Security Administration, State Health Department, State Hospice Organization**, or call the **Medicare Hotline** at (800) 633-4227 to learn about hospice benefits.

If you don't have home access to the Internet, ask your local library or senior center to help you locate any Web site.

Funeral Arrangements and the Grieving Process

Funeral Arrangements and the Grieving Process

*T*o ensure that the wishes of a dying person are carried out and to decrease the level of stress on the family at the time of death, it is helpful for the family to discuss all aspects of the death and all funeral arrangements while the person is still alive. Planning in advance will ensure that the person's wishes are carried out with a minimum of cost. The simpler the service the less expensive it will be, but remember that ritual is important to a bereaved family. Contact funeral homes in your area for specific details.

If your area has a nonprofit memorial association, its volunteers have likely done price comparisons of local funeral homes.

 People often place their funeral instructions in a safe-deposit box that may not be opened until after the funeral. It is better to keep the instructions where they can be easily located and to give a copy to the nearest relative.

Funeral Details to Be Addressed

The more details that are arranged in advance, the easier it is for you, as caregiver, to organize and administer the funeral arrangements. First, choose a company to take charge of all funeral arrangements. Then work with a staff member to decide on the details of the service and burial.

Choosing a Company to Handle Funeral Arrangements

There are three types of organizations that take care of funeral arrangements:

- A traditional funeral home, which can offer a wide range of services

- An immediate disposition company, which will provide either direct burial or direct cremation

- A nonprofit memorial society association

Funeral Details That Can Be Planned in Advance

You will need to make the following decisions:

- What *type of service* is desired—public, private, traditional, religious, or simple memorial

- Whether viewing or visitation of the body prior to the funeral service is desired (and whether the casket should be open or closed)

- Whether the service should include a display of personal photographs and mementos or a video tribute

- Whether the family wants a gathering of relatives and friends to share memories

- Whether there should be a procession from the church or funeral home to the cemetery

- What *type of disposition* of the body is preferred—earth burial, mausoleum entombment, cremation, or burial at sea or in the mountains

- What type of memorial marker is desired

- What *type of casket* is desired—steel, precious metal, or wood; sealed or unsealed; a purchased casket or one rented for the funeral (with a simpler one used for the burial or cremation)

- The clothing desired for the burial

- Whether jewelry is to be buried (not recommended) or removed before burial

- What hair style, makeup, and nail polish is wanted

- Who is to be notified about death: friends, family, employer, the clergy, etc.

- Who will conduct the service and give the eulogy; this might be a member of the clergy, perhaps with personal statements and readings from friends, family, and members of favorite organizations or lodges

- Who the casket bearers will be (avoid people with heart conditions or bad backs and make them honorary casket bearers instead)

- What guest books and prayer cards will be needed

- Which relatives, friends, or business associates need to be notified by phone, letter, or printed notice

- Whether the family has already arranged for ownership of a burial plot, mausoleum crypt, or cremation niche in a cemetery

- What obituary notices should be sent to local papers, hometown papers, and other publications

- What types of flowers are desired for the funeral or memorial service, and where they should be sent afterward (residence, cemetery, nursing home, or church)

- Whether contributions are preferred to flowers and where the contributions are to be sent

- Which musical selections, special Bible passages, poems, literature, tree plantings, or other details are wanted

- Who will send acknowledgment cards to people who gave flowers, food, or other special assistance

Funeral homes are not allowed to charge handling fees on caskets purchased elsewhere and can be fined for refusing to accept them. Contact the State Mortuary and Cemetery Board for details.

Who Can Handle Cremation

- A full-service funeral home

- An immediate disposition company

- A cremation memorial society

An Immediate Disposition Company Will Provide:

- Removal of the deceased from the place of death

- Immediate burial or cremation

- Return of the cremated remains in a container to be placed in a cemetery (or scattered in a special place)

- Help with arrangements if the family wants to scatter the ashes

- Legal paperwork for the death certificate

 Most federal and state regulatory agencies do not impose rules for the spreading of human ashes.

A Funeral Home Will Provide:

All of the above, plus—

- A facility for services, embalming, and the option of viewing the body

- The expertise to help arrange any type of service

Organic and Tissue Donations

Because more than 118,000 Americans are on waiting lists for life-saving organ and tissue transplants, the person in your care may want to be a donor. In some states this can be done by getting the form from the **Department of Motor Vehicles**. Anyone interested in learning about organ donation should start by contacting the **Gift of Hope Organ & Tissue Donor Network** at (888) 307-3668 or by visiting their Web site at www.giftofhope.org. Gift of Hope sponsors a 24/7 donor hotline for professionals at (800) 545-4438.

- Organ and tissue donation has little effect on funeral plans.

- Anyone can be an eye donor, regardless of age or vision.

- Organs that can be donated include the kidneys, heart, pancreas, lungs, liver, and intestines. Tissue such as bone, ligaments, skin, and corneas are also needed.

- There is no age restriction.

- A donor can still have an open-casket funeral since donation does not disfigure the body.

- Organ or tissue donors are still responsible for burial or cremation costs.

- When donating the body for medical education, you still have to pay for embalming and transportation. (The remains are later cremated. They will be disposed of or returned to the family.)

- The estate of the deceased or the family is never charged for the donation.

The Newspaper Obituary

Information needed for the obituary can be gathered in advance with the help of family members. You will need to know—

- Date and place of birth

- Date and place of marriage

- Date death of loved ones

- Employment, education, hobbies

- Civic and public offices held

- Branch of military service, rank, date of discharge

- Church, union, fraternal order memberships

- Names and relations of surviving family members

- Time and place of services

- Memorial contributions

- Charities that should receive memorial donations

Financial Considerations

When deciding on funeral details, state exactly what services you want and then ask for the total price of the services then the itemized version. You want to see what each item costs so you can select only what you want and can afford. Costs can differ dramatically, so make sure you call around and fully understand what you are getting for your money. The **Consumer Affairs** Web site offers a handy pricing checklist: http://www.consumer.ftc.gov/articles/0301-funeral-costs-and-pricing-checklist.

Typical Range of Funeral Costs

Often, the most expensive part of the funeral is the casket, so it is wise to make a selection that is within your budget. Most caskets are purchased directly from the funeral home, but retail casket are available in stores or can be purchased online. You must pay a "professional service" fee that will range anywhere from $695 to $3,000. Ask if the price you get includes this fee or if it is paid separately. The typical range of costs are:

- Immediate burial without any ceremonies—averages $2,700 to $4,000

- Traditional funeral with viewing—can costs up to $10,000 in 2012

- Direct burial or cremations—$1,000–$2,000, plus the cost of the cremation-oriented casket

> **Tip**
>
> Embalming is toxic and use of a steel casket can be costly. A biodegradable shroud (a sheet wrapped around the body) can substitute for a casket, for as little as $40. If you want something sturdier, purchase a biodegradable wood casket, which may cost about $350.

Embalming is necessary if you select a funeral with viewing. However, embalming is not required if you choose direct cremation or immediate burial. Know your legal rights, and shop for the funeral home that makes you feel comfortable. Their concern should be caring for the family, not taking your money.

NOTE These prices are meant to be illustrations. Costs can differ on a regional basis.

Advance Planning

There are many positive reasons for planning funeral and cemetery arrangements in advance. First, important decisions can be made without rushing and without the overwhelming emotional stress and grief that may be present after a death. Advance planning also ensures that the wishes of the deceased will be respected and carried out. Most funeral homes offer "guaranteed" funeral plans that allow services and merchandise to be purchased at today's price.

There are several ways to pay for a funeral, including setting up a personal savings account or arranging for an insurance policy, funeral trust account, or annuity. The advantage of having an insurance policy is that if death occurs before all payments are made, the policy covers the unpaid balance. However, most insurance policies carry significant cancellation penalties if the plan is ever cancelled, and policies will likely be more expensive for older purchasers. Check with your insurance policy provider before you need to use your policy; it could spare you surprises later. Trust accounts are the most liquid and in most states can be cancelled with a full refund including interest. However, if death occurs before all the payments have been made, the survivors must pay the difference. Annuities are similar to trust accounts.

Whichever plan you select, be sure that it—

- Allows you to choose the services you want

- Is transferable if you move out of state or out of the country

- Guarantees that the original price paid, plus the interest, will provide future service at no additional charge. In 2010, a trend enabled insurance companies to charge higher premiums, change terms, and offer no guarantee. You may want to check with a financial planner who won't be trying to sell you a policy for current rules and regulations.

Other Possible Sources of Payment:

- Automobile death insurance benefits

- Crime victims' assistance benefits

- Federal employee benefits

- Funeral fund for members sponsored by fraternal organizations

- Social Security (a very small death benefit)

- Union death fund

- Veteran's allowance

> **NOTE** In cases of poverty, seek advice from a member of the clergy, a rabbi, or a funeral director.

Information That Will Be Needed After Death

Many facts can be gathered in a person's lifetime and recorded in a simple Estate Planner. Keep this little booklet or form (available from most funeral homes, some attorneys, and stationery stores) in a safe place and let the family know where it is located.

Be sure you have telephone numbers for the following people so you can reach them easily:

- Accountant

- Attorney

- Business associates

- Clergy

- Doctor

- Employees

- Employer

- Estate executor or trustee

- Family

- Financial advisor

- Friends

- Funeral home where the funeral is pre-planned

- Health representative, if other than you

- Tax preparer

Financial Information to Record in Your Estate Planner

In an estate planning booklet or informal list, keep clear records of the following information, complete with account numbers, addresses, telephone numbers, and the location of the documents:

- Investments, their amounts, and brokers

- Annuities

- Bank checking and savings accounts

- Life insurance policy numbers

- Medicare and supplemental insurance

- Military service and veterans' benefits

- Mortgages and liabilities

- Pension plans, profit-sharing, Keogh plans, and IRAs

- Real estate holdings

- Safe-deposit box location and key

- Social Security card and number and the date benefits began, if applicable

- Workers compensation, if applicable

- List of motor vehicles owned and location of titles

When a person dies, his *estate*—all the stuff he owned while alive (home, car, cash, etc.)—will be responsible for paying his debts. Whatever is left over is passed along to his heirs, as dictated by the terms of his will, if he has one. If he does not have a will, the intestacy (inheritance) laws of the state he resides in (visit **www.mystatewill.com**) will determine how his estate will be distributed.

If, however, he dies broke or there isn't enough money left over to pay unsecured debts—things like credit cards, medical bills, personal loans—then his estate is declared *insolvent*, and his creditors (those he owes) will get nothing.

There are, however, a couple of exceptions that could make children legally responsible for their parent's unsecured debt after the parent passes away. These are if the son or daughter is a joint holder on a credit card account that has a balanced owing, or if they co-signed on a loan with the deceased person. Visit **www.SavvySenior.org** for more information.

Survivors' Benefits

Carefully check all life and casualty insurance and death benefits. Check on income for survivors from a credit union, trade union, fraternal organization, the military, and the Social Security Administration. Some debts and installment payments may carry insurance clauses that will cancel them. Consult with creditors if there will be a delay in payments and ask for more time.

Social Security Benefits

The widow, dependent widower, children, and dependent parents of an insured person may be eligible for monthly survivors' payments. (They usually don't start for about six weeks). However, Social Security benefits are not paid automatically. To apply, you will need the following documents:

- Birth certificate of the deceased

- Marriage certificate

- Birth certificates of survivors (under 22 years of age if they are full-time college students; under 18 if they are not)

- Proof of widow's or widower's age, if 62 or older

- Proof of termination of any preceding marriage

- Record of income for the preceding year

The surviving spouse or minor children may also receive a modest one-time death benefit. Ask your Social Security office for help in filling out your claims.

A personalized **Social Security report**, which outlines benefits, earnings history, and other useful information can be obtained by calling (800) 772-1213; for TTY (800)-325-0778. Or, go online to: www.ssa.gov/myaccount.

If you have an email address, you can obtain an electronic estimate of Social Security retirement and disability benefits, as well as benefits paid to the survivors, by signing on to the Web site www.ssa.gov. It will not include a complete earnings history. You must know the person's name, Social Security number, date of birth, place of birth, and mother's maiden name.

The Experience of Grief

Grieving is a natural and important process that helps us avoid depression and psychological problems later. The stages of grief are different for all of us—and the time it takes to pass through them varies. (In general, one must experience at least one set of seasons and holidays without a loved one, but often the grieving process takes much longer than that.)

As you grieve, you may experience such intense and conflicting emotions that you feel you are going crazy. This happens to many people. However, by recognizing the common stages of grief, you can handle feelings that might otherwise be alarming. Remember, the grieving process is natural and, ultimately, will restore balance to your life.

These are some common stages (from Granger Westburg and E. Kubler-Ross) in the grieving process:

- Shock and numbness—usually the first stage, which can last from a few days to several months

- Emotional release—as shock wears off

- Depression—loneliness and isolation

- Symptoms of distress—taking on the symptoms of the illness

- Disorganization and anxiety—confusion and an inability to concentrate, causing feelings of panic

- Hostility—anger at medical staff, clergy, friends, "why didn't you do more?"

- Guilt—remembering the negatives to offset the beauty and blame

- Hesitancy to renew normal activities—the fear of returning to regular activities; of feeling sad at hear a familiar song

- Healing of memories—a time of reaching out, even fearfully, to embrace fully all that has happened and to accept these life changes

- The acceptance of one's new role—Realizing that the cycle of life continues; the bereaved person can finally shed the cloak of grief and take on the role of peace

 NOTE It is helpful to deal with grief by being around people who have gone through the same experience. Most communities have grief support groups through churches, synagogues, county mental health departments, hospice, and other nonprofit organizations.

Serious Warning Signs

Seek professional counseling if you or a family member develops a medical condition in reaction to profound feelings of loss or:

- Feels strong hostility

- Loses all emotional feeling

- Begins using alcohol or drugs

- Feels happiness instead of a sense of loss

- Withdraws from all friendships

- Is profoundly depressed or suicidal

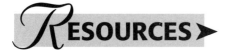

RESOURCES ►

AARP
(800) 424-3410
www.aarp.org/relationships/grief-loss/

Funeral Consumers Alliance
33 Patchen Road
South Burlington, VT 05403
(800) 865-8300
www.funerals.org
Provides information about alternatives for funeral or non-funeral dispositions; can refer you to individual societies in the state of your choice.

The Funeral Service Center
www.funeral.com
Gift of Hope Organ & Tissue Donor Network
425 Spring Lake Drive
Itasca, IL 60143
(888) 307-3668
(630) 758-2600
(630) 758-2601 (fax)
info@giftofhope.org
www.giftofhope.org
Web site provides a Crisis, Grief, & Healing Discussion Page.

Grief And Healing Discussion Page
www.webhealing.com
Offers a discussion group on the Internet for people dealing with grief.

Last Acts
www.lastacts.org
Comprehensive Web site with links to resources for end-of-life care.

Grieving.com
http://forums.grieving.com/

GriefShare
PO Box 1739
Wake Forest, NC 27588
(800) 395-5755
info@griefshare.org
www.griefshare.org
Offers seminars and support groups throughout the United States and Canada.

Grief Recovery Institute Guidance Center
www.tributes.com/grief_recovery_center

The Grief Recovery Kit
www.griefrecoverykit.com
A young person's guide through grief.

Public Reference Branch
Federal Trade Commission
http://www.consumer.ftc.gov/articles/pdf-0056-funerals.pdf
Provides access to "Facts for Consumers: Funerals A Consumer Guide." Also visit: http://www.consumer.ftc.gov/articles/0070-shopping-funeral-services

National Funeral Directors Association
http://nfda.org/public.html
The loss of a loved one is one of the most difficult experiences of life. Resources on this Web site can help those mourning the loss of a loved one with ways to cope with their grief, ideas for memorial services and funerals, and a way to locate their local NFDA Member Funeral Director. NFDA Member Funeral Directors abide by a professional code of conduct that ensures they care for your loved one with the compassion and respect you expect.

Regional Pathology and Autopsy Services (Nationwide)
http://www.regional-pathology.com/families/
When a loved one dies, it is a time of great upheaval and stress. You may feel overwhelmed by all the questions surrounding your loved one's death, or you might simply want closure and peace of mind. An autopsy can help you understand the circumstances that led to the loss of your loved one, as well as any genetic or inherited diseases that may continue on to future generations.

Write or call your local state **Mortuary and Cemetery Board** or your **State Funeral Directors Association** for information on funerals.

If you don't have home access to the Internet, ask your local library or senior center to help you locate any Web site.

Part Three: Additional Resources

Common Abbreviations

ABI – acquired brain injury

Acute MI – heart attack

ADA – Americans with Disabilities Act

ADL – activities of daily living

AFO – ankle-foot orthotics

ALF – assisted living facility

ASHD – arteriosclerotic heart disease

BC – blood culture

BID – 2 times per day (approximately 8 and 8 as medication times)

BP – blood pressure

BRP – bathroom privileges

BS – blood sugar

C&S – culture and sensitivity

CA – cancer/carcinoma

CABG – coronary artery bypass graft

CBC – complete blood count

CBR – complete bed rest

CCU – coronary care unit

CHF – congestive heart failure

CNS – central nervous system

COPD – chronic obstructive pulmonary disease

CPR – cardiopulmonary resuscitation

Crt – critical

Cs – case

CSF – cerebrospinal fluid

CVA – cerebral vascular accident

CVD – cerebral vascular disease

DM – diabetes mellitus

DME – durable medical equipment

DNR – do not resuscitate

DRG – diagnosis related group

Dx – diagnosis

ED – emergency department

EEG – electroencephalogram recording of the brain's electrical activity

EKG/ECG – electrocardiogram recording of the heart's electrical activity

EP – evoked potential

FBS – fasting blood sugar, or the amount of glucose in the blood when a person has not eaten for 12 hours

FX – fracture

GCS – Glasgow coma scale

GTT – glucose tolerance test to determine a person's ability to metabolize glucose

HC – home care

HHA – a home health agency providing home health services

HS – hour of sleep (medication time)

I&O – record of food and liquid taken in and waste eliminated

ICU – intensive care unit for special monitoring of the acutely ill

IV – intravenous line to drip fluids and blood products into the bloodstream

LOC – loss of consciousness

MCD – Medicaid

MCR – Medicare

MRI – magnetic resonance imaging

Neuro – neurologist

NPO – nothing by mouth

NSAID's – non-steroidal anti-inflammatory drugs

OBS – organic brain syndrome, an injury or disorder that interferes with normal brain function

OR – operating room

OT – occupational therapy or occupational therapist

PO – by mouth

Psych – psychologist

PT – physical therapy or physical therapist

QID – 4 times per day (approximately 9–1–5–9 as medication times)

RBC – red blood count

RN – nurse

ROM – range of motion

RR – respiratory rate

RT – recreational therapy

Rx – prescription

SLP – speech-language pathologist

SNF – skilled nursing facility

SOB – shortness of breath

SS or SSA – Social Security or Social Security Administration

SSI/SSDI – supplemental security income or disability income

ST – Speech therapist or speech therapy

Sx – symptoms

TBI – traumatic brain injury

TIA – transient ischemic attack

TID – 3 times per day (approximately 9–1–6 as medication times)

TPN – total parenteral nutrition (intravenous)

TPR – temperature, pulse, respiration

TX – treatment

U/A – urine analysis

VEP – visual evoked potential

VNS – visiting nurse service

WBC – white blood count

Common Specialists

Allergist/Immunologist
Disorders of the immune system

Anesthesiologist
Pain relief during and after surgery

Audiologist
Hearing disorders

Cardiologist
Conditions of the heart, lungs, and blood vessels

Chiropodist
Minor foot ailments such as corns and bunions

Colon and Rectal Surgeon
Diseases of the intestinal tract

Dentist
Teeth and gums

Dermatologist
Skin, hair, and nails

Endocrinologist
Hormonal problems including thyroid disorders

Forensic Psychiatrist
Behavior assessment for legal purposes

Gastroenterologist
Digestive system, stomach, liver, bowels, and gallbladder

Geriatric Psychiatrist
Emotional disorders of elderly persons

Geriatrician
Disorders common to elderly persons

Gynecologist
Female reproductive system

Hematologist
Diseases of the blood, spleen, and lymph glands

Internist
Primary care of common illnesses, both long term and emergency

Nephrologist
Kidney diseases and disorders

Neurologist
Brain and nervous system disorders

Nurse Practitioner
Provides preventive and medical health care in association with a physician

Oncologist
All cancers

Ophthalmologist
Care and surgery of the eyes

Optician
Fitting and making of eyeglasses and contact lenses

Optometrist
Basic eye care

Oral Maxillofacial Surgeon
Surgery involving the teeth, gums, and jaw

Orthopedist
Surgery involving joints, bones, and muscles

Orthotist
Nonmedical specialist in the measurement, sizing, and preparation of foot padding pieces

Osteopath (DO)
General medicine with emphasis on the promotion of health through the hands-on manipulation of the muscles, tendons, and joints

Otolaryngologist
Head and neck surgeon

Pharmacist
Medications specialist; provider of physician and patient education

Podiatrist
Foot care

Psychiatrist
Rehabilitation assessment and planning

Psychiatrist (MD)
Emotional, mental, or addictive disorders

Psychologist (MA or PhD)
Assessment and care of emotional or mental disorders

Pulmonologist
Diseases of lungs and airways

Rheumatologist
Diseases of joints and connective tissue (arthritis)

Urogynecologist
Specialist in problems that affect a woman's control of bladder and other pelvic organs.

Urologist
Urinary system and the male reproductive system

Glossary

A

Activities of daily living (ADL): personal hygiene, bathing, dressing, grooming, toileting, feeding, and transferring

Acute: state of illness that comes on suddenly and may be of short duration

Adult day care: centers that have a supervised environment where seniors can be with others

Advance directive: a legal document that states a person's health care preferences in writing while that person is competent and able to make such decisions

Ambulatory: able to walk with little or no assistance

Amnesia: complete or partial loss of memory

Analgesics: medications used to relieve pain

Antibiotics: a group of drugs used to combat infection

Anus: the opening of the rectum

Anxiety: a state of discomfort, dread, and foreboding with physical symptoms such as rapid breathing and heart rate, tension, jitteriness, and muscle aches

Apathy: a condition in which the person shows little or no emotion

Aromatherapy: use of essential oils of various plants to treat symptoms of diseases, improve sleep, and reduce stress by inducing relaxation

Artificial life-support systems: the use of respirators, tube feeding, intravenous (IV) feeding, and other means to replace natural and vital functions, such as breathing, eating, and drinking

Assessment: the process of analyzing a person's condition

Assisted living: residential housing for seniors offering independence, choice of services, and assistance with Activities of Daily living, including meals and housekeeping

Assistive devices: any tools that are designed, fabricated, and/or adapted to assist a person in performing a particular task, e.g., cane, walker, show chair

Assistive technology: a term used to describe all of the tools, products and devices, from the simplest to the most complex, which can make a particular function easier to perform

Atrophy: the wasting away of muscles or brain tissue

↝ B

Bedpan: a container into which a person urinates and defecates while in bed

Blood pressure: the pressure of the blood on the walls of the blood vessels and arteries

Body language: gestures that serve as a form of communication

Body mechanics: proper use and positioning of the body to do work and avoid strain and injury

↝ C

Calorie: the measure of the energy the body gets from various foods

Cataract: a condition (often found in the elderly) in which the lens of the eye become opaque

Catheter: a rubber tube for collecting urine from a person who has become incontinent

Chronic: refers to a state or condition that lasts 6 months or longer

Cognition: high-level functions carried out by the human brain, including comprehension and use of speech, visual perception and construction, calculation ability, attention (information processing), memory, and executive functions such as planning, problem-solving, and self-monitoring

Cognitive rehabilitation: techniques used to improve the functioning of individuals whose cognition is impaired because of physical trauma or disease

Colostomy: a temporary or permanent surgical procedure that creates an artificial opening through the abdominal wall into a part of the large bowel through which feces can leave the body

Congregate living: a type of independent living in which elderly people can live in their own apartments but have meals, laundry, transportation, and housekeeping services available

Conservator: a person given the power to take over and protect the interests of one who is incompetent

Constipation: difficulty having bowel movements

Contracture: shortening or tightening of the tissue around a joint so that the person loses the ability to move easily

D

Decubitus ulcer: pressure sore; bedsore

Defecate: to have a bowel movement

Defibrillator: a device that uses and electrical current to restore or regulate a stopped or disorganized heartbeat

Dehydration: loss of normal body fluid, sometimes caused by vomiting and severe diarrhea

Delusions: beliefs that are firmly held despite proof that they are false

Dementia: a progressive decline in mental functions

Depression: a psychiatric condition that can be moderate or severe and cause feelings of sadness and emptiness

Diuretics: drugs that help the body get rid of fluids

Draw sheet: a sheet folded widthwise to position under someone in bed to keep the linen clean and aid in transfers

Durable Power of Attorney: a legal document that authorizes another to act as one's agent and is "durable" because it remains in effect in case the person becomes disabled or mentally incompetent

Durable Power of Attorney for Health Care Decisions: a legal document that lets a person name someone else to make health care decisions after the person has become disabled or mentally incompetent and is unable to make those decisions

Dysphagia: difficulty with or abnormal swallowing

E

Edema: an abnormal swelling in legs, ankles, hands, or abdomen that occurs because the body is retaining fluids

Estate planning: a process of planning for the present and future use of a person's assets

∾ F

Foot drop: a condition of weakness in the muscles of the foot and ankle, caused by poor nerve conduction, which interferes with a person's ability to flex the ankle and walk with a normal heel–toe pattern; the toes touch the ground before the heel, causing the person to trip or lose balance

Foster care: a care arrangement in which a person lives in a private home with a primary caregiver and 4 or 5 other people

∾ G

Gait: the manner in which a person walks

Geriatric: refers to people 65 or older

Guardian: the one who is designated to have protective care of another person or of that person's property

∾ H

Hallucination: false perceptions of things that are not really there

Heimlich maneuver: a method for clearing the airway of a choking person

Hospice: a program that allows a dying person to remain at home while receiving professionally supervised care

∾ I

Incontinence: involuntary discharge of urine or feces

Intravenous (IV): the delivery of fluids, medications, or nutrients into a vein

Involved: a term used to describe the side of the body most affected by a disease, operation, or medical condition

∾ L

Laxative: a substance taken to increase bowel movements and prevent constipation

M

Mechanical lift: a machine used to lift a person from one place to another

Medic-Alert®: bracelet identification system linked to a 24-hour service that provides full information in the case of an emergency

Medicaid: a public health program that uses state and federal funds to pay certain medical and hospital expenses of those having low income or no income, with benefits that vary from state to state

Medicare: the federal health insurance program for people 65 or older and for certain people under 65 who are disabled

N

Nutrition: a process of giving the body the key nutrients it needs for proper body function

O

Occupational therapy: therapy that focuses on the activities of daily living such as personal hygiene, bathing, dressing, grooming, toileting, and feeding

Ombudsman: a person who helps residents of a retirement or health care facility with such problems as quality of care, food, finances, medical care, residents rights, and other concerns; these services are confidential and free

Oral hygiene: the process of keeping the mouth clean

P

Paralysis: loss or impairment of voluntary movement of a group of muscles

Paranoia: a mental disorder characterized by delusions (often the belief that one is being persecuted)

Paraplegic: one who is paralyzed in (usually) the lower half of the body

Passive suicide: killing oneself through indirect action or inaction, such as no longer taking life-prolonging medications

Pathogen: a disease-causing microorganism

Physical therapy: the process of relearning walking, balancing, and transfers

Posey: a vest-like restraint used to keep a person from getting out of bed

Positioning: placing a person in a position that allows functional activity and minimizes the danger of faulty posture that could cause pressure sores, impaired breathing, and shrinking of muscles and tendons

Power of Attorney for Health Care: providing another person with the authority to make health care decisions

Pressure sore: a breakdown of the skin caused by prolonged pressure in one spot; a bed sore; decubitus ulcer

Prognosis: a forecast of what is likely to happen when an individual contracts a particular disease or condition

Prone: lying facedown

Prosthesis: an artificial body part, such as a tooth, an eye, a breast, leg, arm, hand, or foot

Q

Quadriplegia: paralysis of both the upper and lower parts of the body from the neck down

R

Range of motion (ROM): the extent of possible passive (movement by another person) movement in a joint

Rehabilitation: after a disabling injury or disease, restoration of a person's maximum physical, mental, vocational, social, and spiritual potential

Respite care: short-term care that allows a primary caregiver time off from his or her responsibilities

Rigidity: a tightness or increase in muscle tone at rest or throughout the entire range of motion of a limb, which may be felt as stiffness by the patient

S

Sedatives: medications used to calm a person

Shock: a state of collapse resulting from reduced blood volume and/or blood pressure caused by burns, severe injury, pain, or an emotional blow

Sitz bath: a bath in which only the hips and buttocks are immersed into water or a medicated solution

Speech therapy: the treatment of disorders of communication, including expressive language, writing, and reading and communication required for activities of daily living

Stroke: sudden loss of function of a part of the brain due to interference in its blood supply, usually by hemorrhage or blood clotting

Supine: lying on one's back

Support groups: groups of people who get together to share common experiences and help one another cope

Symptom: sign of a disease or disorder that helps in diagnosis

ॐ T

Tracheotomy: surgical procedure to make an opening in a person's windpipe to aid in breathing

Tranquilizers: a class of drugs used to calm a person and control certain emotional disturbances

Transfer: movements from one position to another, for example, from bed to chair, wheelchair to car, etc.

Transfer belt: a device placed around the waist of a disabled person and used to secure the person while walking; gait belt

Transfer board (Sliding Board): polished wooden or plastic board used to slide a person when moving from one place to another, for example, bed to wheelchair or commode

Trapeze: a metal bar suspended over a bed to help a person raise up or move

ॐ U

Urinal: a container used by a bedridden male for urinating

Urinalysis: a laboratory test of urine

ॐ V

Vaginal douche: a procedure to cleanse or medicate a woman's vagina by sending a stream of water into the vaginal opening

Vital signs: life signs such as blood pressure, breathing, and pulse

Void: to urinate; pass water

ॐ W

Will: a legal document that states how to dispose of a person's property after death according to that person's wishes

Index

preparing for, 358
principles of, 359–363
questions to ask, 359
Hospital, protecting person's best
            interests in, 40–42
Hospital bed, 138
Hospital-type equipment, specialized, 150
Hostility of caregiver, 177
House sharing, 13
Hydraulic lift, 139
Hypnosis, 264
Hypothermia, 327–328
    signs of, 327–328

Ideal caregiver, checklist, 11
Immediate disposition company, 369
Income tax, 95–100
    deductions, 97–99
    dependent, qualification as, 95–96
    funeral expenses, 99
    medical expense deductions, 97–98
    tax credits, for elderly/disabled, 96–97
    year-end tax tips, 99–100
Incontinence, 217–218
Individual practice associations plans, 83
Infection control, 221–225
    body fluids, disposal of, 224
    cleaning techniques, 221–224
    hand-washing by caregiver, 222
    laundry, soiled, 222–223
    odors caused by bacteria, 224–225
    sterilization, 223–224
        wet heat sterilization, 223
    wheelchair, patient propelling, 222
Information needed after death, 374–377
Infusion equipment, 150
Inhalers, 150
Instrumental activities of daily living, 6
Internet, 258–259
Isolation, sense of, in caregiver, 176

Kitchen, 125–126
    comfort/convenience measures, 125–126
    safety measures, 125

Lack of appetite, 231–232
Lap board, 240
Laundry, soiled, 222–223
Lease, signing, 18
Leaving facility, rights of residents, 19–20
Leg problems, 207
Level of care needed, 5–7
Licensed practical nurse, 59
Lift chair, 139
Listening aids, 145
Living trust, 93
Living will, 93, 251–254 109, 271, 358
Locating personal assistant, 57–58
Long-range planning, 28
Long term planning for caregiver, 184–190

Massage therapy, 242–243, 310
Meals on Wheels, 87, 229
Mechanical lift, transfers using, 348–349
Medicaid, 16, 62, 16, 20, 74–78, 101–103
    asset transfers, 74, 102–103
    common aspects of, 75–76
    services not covered, 76–77
Medical decisions, sharing in, 27–31
Medical equipment, 138–144
Medical expense tax deductions, 97–98
Medicare, 16, 20, 52–53, 68–74, 137, 361–362
    eligibility, 68–69
    Part B insurance, 72
    Part D, Prescription Drug Plan, 70–71
    payments by, 69–70
    services not covered, 72
    Supplemental Insurance, 71–74
Medication, schedule (sample form), 166
Medications
    appealing health maintenance organization
            decisions, 86
    questions to ask doctor, 33–34
    recording/managing, 165–168
    travel with, 275
Medigap, 16, 73–74
Meditation, 183–184, 264
Mental health treatment, 38
Mobility aids, 142–144
Motivation, 309–310